# HOW WE BECAME
## BREAST CANCER
# THRIVERS

### Our hindsight can be your foresight

ISBN 978-0-9768995-0-1

PUBLISHER:     Thrivers Publishing L.L.C.
                       P.O. Box 2040
                       Lebanon, MO  65536

Cover book design by Stacie Marshall, Hill Design Co.

Printed in the United States of America

# HOW WE BECAME
## BREAST CANCER
# THRIVERS

### Our hindsight can be your foresight

Beverly Vote,
PUBLISHER OF THE BREAST CANCER WELLNESS MAGAZINE
and 44 Stories from Her Breast Cancer Thriving Friends
Now Living with Conviction, Clarity, Passion and Purpose

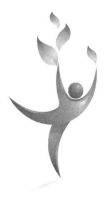

"There is a light in this world... a healing spirit much stronger
than any darkness we may encounter.
We sometimes lose sight of this force...
where there is suffering and too much pain.
And suddenly the spirit will emerge,
through ordinary people and answer in extraordinary ways.
God speaks in the silence of the heart when we listen."

*~Mother Teresa*

# Show Me
# the Way Out

Mary Ann thought she had everything going her way
Until breast cancer was to change her every day.
In anguish, Mary Ann cries out, her pleas full of doubt.
She was in a dark hole with no light to show her way out.

She thought she had hope when a doctor walked by.
Why didn't he understand her tear filled cry?
He wrote her a prescription and went on his scheduled way.
But her hopes and her direction were still in dark dismay.

Again, Mary Ann cries out, her pleas full of doubt.
This time a priest nearby heard her shout.
He walked to the hole Mary Ann was in.
I hear your cries, I will pray for your sin.
Bless you my child, he had to say,
And gave three Hail Marys to anoint her way.

Once again, Mary Ann cries out, her pleas full of doubt.
Quietly a stranger responds,
I know your fears inside and out.
I know the secrets hidden within.
I know too well this hole that you are in.

The stranger jumped without hesitation
Into the hole filled with so much tribulation.
Bewildered, Mary Ann cries out, her pleas full of doubt.
What have you done, why are you here?
I appreciate your grace,
But now we are both in this dark, dark place.

Shhhsssh, says the stranger to Mary Ann.
I hear your cries, your pleas full of doubt.
I have been here myself, as a survivor showed me,
I will show you the way out.

*–Beverly Vote*

# Contents

*To survive is our starting point.*
*To thrive is our original design.*

*~Beverly Vote*

# Introduction

In these 44 chapters are messages from breast cancer thrivers who candidly share their beliefs and experiences that helped change them from being scared and helpless to being empowered.

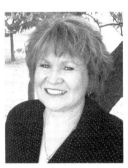

Beverly Vote

You will read about choice, advocacy, advanced stages and recurrence of breast cancer, divorce after breast cancer, new careers, new love, life lessons, and life purpose. Many chapters include messages how their Faith and a higher spiritual power played a role in how to thrive, and others learned how to believe in themselves and that their life mattered. Some of us believe that our diagnosis of breast cancer wasn't meant to be a death sentence as projected by the medical experts, but a calling to heal not only our body but to heal our life and be the person we were created to be. For me, the breast cancer experience was a disguised learning lesson and a spiritual awakening and transformational tool to help deliver me from my unhealthy beliefs and thoughts about my feminine worthiness.

We are grateful because we know, we really know, we are stronger because of the experience and how we look at life and how we face daily challenges are with a broader perspective and with a stronger understanding of who we are.

I am Beverly Vote. I am a Thriver! I am grateful.

# 1.
# Everything Happens for a Reason

## BY JUDY BAKER

*Judy Baker is an 8 year breast cancer thriver. She has a Master's degree in education, which she uses every day in her career as a self-employed investment advisor and retirement planner. Judy is 61 years old and her goal is to do whatever it takes to get the most out of each and every day.*

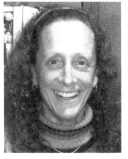

Every breast cancer thriver has a story to tell. Mine is not better, just different—as they all are. My goal is that by writing this, at least one person will feel more hope, have more balance in their life, be more in tune with their body, and in general, appreciate life a little more. I hope that my contribution will help someone else to thrive.

My own story began in 1996, at age 47, with a diagnosis of DCIS—ductal carcinoma insitu in one breast. After a biopsy, it was treated with radiation and tamoxifen. But there was a recurrence three and one half years later, which was treated with another biopsy. After a third occurrence, my doctor recommended a mastectomy of that breast, because of the strong potential that the next episode would be invasive. He said that there was no medical reason to remove the other breast. It took a few days of soul searching, but I came to the conclusion that if both were removed, I probably wouldn't have to deal with it all again. So in August of 2002 I had both breasts removed. They were fun while I had them, but they had served their purpose. I nursed two babies straight to regular drinking cups. What else could I ask for?!

I also chose not to have breast reconstruction. It just wasn't right for me. Please know that I truly believe that each woman has the right to make that decision for herself. One person's choice is not right for everyone.

I have never regretted either decision, and in fact, have been relieved many times over. I was quite small breasted before surgery, so now I'm just flatter! My surgical nurse, a friend of mine, told me later that she kidded with my doctor that the bandages made me look larger than I was before surgery. She has called me on my surgery anniversary date to remind me of that. Thanks Lisa!

So that's my story in a nutshell. But it's just the spark that lit my strong need to thrive. I don't think that a day goes by that I am not reminded of how precious life is. I know that my dear friend Gretchen felt that way too. She was first diagnosed with breast cancer in 1990. She then fought it on and off for fifteen years. But Gretchen had a dream. So when she found out, about five years ago, that she didn't have much time left—at age 62, her breast cancer had come back with a vengeance—she passed her dream on to a few of her close friends. I feel blessed that I was one of them.

Before her death, Gretchen had a vision of a Dragon Boat team in the Mid-Ohio Valley. That's the area of southeast Ohio around Marietta, where two rivers meet—the Muskingum and the Ohio. From the day Gretchen first learned of Dragon Boating, she envisioned our town (Marietta) being ideal for the sport. Just before her death, she attended our first organizational meeting, the MOV'n Dragons was established. Gretchen made the initial contribution. Then, friends and family donated gifts to her memory, to the Marietta Community Foundation, allowing us to purchase the boat, paddles and life jackets. Our boat is 45 feet long, weighs about 500 pounds and holds 20 paddlers. A drummer/coach sits in front, keeping the strokes in unison, and a steers person stands in the back, keeping us on course. Our boat is named "Gretchen's Phoenix", and every time we paddle I can feel Gretchen there with us.

Originating in China over 2000 years ago, Dragon Boating was a part of a celebration of the revered dragon, which people believed would ensure them with bountiful crops and good health. Adopted by sports enthusiasts as a rigorous sport world-wide since then, in the late 1980's it was prescribed as a physical regimen for breast cancer thrivers to overcome the side effects of surgery, and to provide the support and friendship of other thrivers. Today, Dragon Boating is a world-wide sport with races and festivals celebrating wellness and fitness for all participants.

If, ten years ago, someone had told me that I would be paddling a Dragon Boat, I would have laughed very hard. Two reasons—I'm scared to death of the water and, I have never in my life participated in a group sport. Well, I guess we surprise ourselves sometimes. The experience has been the most exciting and rewarding one that I have ever had over this length of time.

We are starting our fourth summer now, which of course, is our busy time. The first two summers saw the development of our core group. We got to know each other and have fun whenever we got together. Over the third summer and now into this summer, we have started to train and be more competitive. Each summer our group grows, which is rewarding in itself.

Last summer was the first time we actually participated in Dragon Boat races and were part of two Dragon Boat Festivals. I can now say with conviction that Dragon Boating is in my blood! The first Festival that we attended was in Toledo, Ohio. Only ten of us were able to go, so we joined up with another group to fill the boat. We were all either thrivers or supporters.

It started raining early the morning of the races. We all planned on getting drenched. In the first nine heats everyone did get soaked. But just before our first race, the clouds parted and the sun actually came out! It was a sign of things to come.

In our first race, we came in second - a very satisfying result since we had to do the race twice after the three other boats blew off course and went into the wrong lanes, causing all four boats to have to start all over again. So we had to paddle back to the start, and race the 500 meters to the finish—two times. It was exhausting, but the adrenalin that runs through you in a race is extremely invigorating. It was also quite encouraging that the folks (mostly guys) who sponsored the boat we were in, and paddled with us were VERY muscular. We MOVED through that water!

The second race was not quite so rewarding. We came in fourth. Water and wind conditions had changed. No excuses, we were last.

Something kicked in for all of us on our third and final race. We were psyched, excited and full of spit and vinegar. As we approached the starting line, I yelled back: "this is it guys—let's show 'em!" And we did. Our coach and drummer at the front of the boat yelled commands louder than ever. Our steers person in the back, knew just what he had to do to keep us on course, and he did it beautifully (even after being hit by another boat near the end of the race). Our power strokes were executed with energy and determination.

Out of nowhere, our Toledo teammates started chanting in deep resonant voices, "DIG! DIG! DIG!", to the metronome of the drum beat. For 500 meters we dug deeper than we ever had before. As we crossed the finish line, I dared to look to our left where I expected to see the other three boats. They were behind us! WE WON! Not just a trophy (which we did get by the way), but a taste of what can be achieved when a team works as one.

It's very hard to describe the feeling you have when something like that happens. All I can say is "What a rush!" It was like nothing I'd ever felt before. All of those hours of practice; all of the aching muscles and blisters; all of the wise cracks we exchanged while at paddling practice; all of the friendships we established; all of the sharing of our lives' experiences came to one moment of total exhilaration - not so much because we won the race, but because of what we had all put into that race that made us so successful.

As soon as I realized what we had accomplished, a lump came to my throat and tears to my eyes. Thank you Gretchen, for your courage. Thank you teammates, for all of your work and enthusiasm. Most of all, thank you Joe, my husband, for unending support and participation in MOV'n Dragons.

Our second festival was in Cleveland, Ohio. This time we had a full boat of MOV'n Dragon team members. Again we participated in three races, two of them against the Akron, Ohio team. A little background - Akron was our mentor team. They even came down to Marietta with their boat to practice and "race" with us. We learned so much from their generosity in wanting to help us. So we almost felt guilty when we beat them at the Cleveland Festival - not once, but twice. I think that what we will all remember most about that day was what happened after we finished the last race. We walked along the dock to the steps leading to the gathering area. The Akron team members were all standing in two lines facing each other at the top of the steps, with paddles crossed overhead forming an arch above the walkway we came through—in tribute to us! There wasn't a dry eye in the house. Adrenalin was still pumping, and emotions were running high. We all felt the sense of total accomplishment from following a dream to its conclusion, and achieving things we never would have imagined possible.

We won all three races that day, and now we have quite a legacy to carry forward. But we're up to it. Though we all work very hard practicing, we have lots of fun too. And isn't that what life is all about?

I love being part of Dragon Boating. It lets me express my zest for life by being a part of a dynamic, fun loving, life loving group. It fits! Being part of the Dragon Boat experience helps me release the thriving spirit within me. The team spirit helps me dig deep within myself every time and helps me keep my thriver energy going strong. Life is important and sharing it with others who also feel passionate about thriving is exhilarating.

Sometimes I wonder why cancer happened to me. I don't have that answer, but I know that if I had not been through that experience, I probably would never have had the Dragon Boat experience. There's nothing I could imagine that would ever come close to what I've gained from being part of the MOV'n Dragons. We are all living Gretchen's dream, but it has become our dream too.

I'm a true believer in "everything happens for a reason". No need to say more.

# 2.

# From Survivor to Thriver: Life at a Higher Level

## BY REV. KAREN BALDWIN

*Rev. Baldwin is an Interfaith Minster, teacher and writer. The story of her work in KwaZulu-Natal, "High Hopes and Other Illusions: Lost and Found in Africa" is due in 2011. Karen lives in Taos, New Mexico where she maintains a spiritual counseling practice, facilitates dream groups, and mentors individuals through life changes. To learn more, visit www.ChangeHealGrow.me or email Karen@ChangeHealGrow.me.*

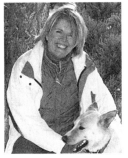

When the phone rang that mid-November afternoon, I wasn't expecting what I was about to hear. All along my doctor had said, "It's probably nothing," and I believed her. When she said "carcinoma" I quit listening and went stumbling, in absolute dread, into the darkness of my interior. My life replayed through my mind as if I were approaching death. Every mistake I had ever made, every sweet moment I wanted to feel again, and every dream that I had left undone, took center stage. I wasn't ready to give up on life.

"Karen, will that be okay?" she asked, jolting me back into the moment. No! Nothing is okay, I thought. The bottom had just dropped out of my world. Life as I knew it, had just ended, and my choices felt limited. I could either crawl into a hole and get caught in the downward spiral of being a victim, or I could agree to see her the next day to discuss treatment options.

Along with the devastating news that cancer was inhabiting my breast came the feeling of being trapped in my body. I felt contaminated and wanted to crawl out of my skin. I also felt betrayed by my body and my spiritual beliefs. For twenty-three years I had subscribed to the concept that I create my own circumstances through the energy of cause and effect. Having already experienced many examples of how my life played out according to the thoughts on which I dwelled, I was efficient at monitoring my mental activity.

It was inconceivable to me that I had created this crisis—being a cancer patient had never even crossed my mind. Cancer doesn't run in my family. I eat a healthy diet, don't smoke and rarely drink. I'd done everything right. It seemed as though I were being punished for some horrible, mysterious mistake, something I would never have an opportunity to correct. I was angry, confused and terrified.

But there was no time to waste sorting out what cancer meant in the scheme of my life, or how it was connected to my spirituality. There were decisions to be made, and hesitation could be fatal. For the next month I lived to go to the doctor. I had a lumpectomy that failed to remove all the cancer, followed by visits with a variety of specialists to discuss the pros and cons of radiation (considering the fact that I have a heart condition). At the end of the month I had collected an assortment of further treatment possibilities.

Moments of peace were rare during that time. They came only in the first few moments after I woke in the morning, before my memory kicked in to remind me of the cancer growing in my body. Lapsing into excruciating fear and rage, I moved through my days extremely short-tempered, venting my anger on anyone who dared to cross me. Unleashed from my previously calm and gentle mannerisms, neither my partner nor I knew how to handle my new emotional extremes. At night, exhausted from my strong feelings and the endless doctor appointments, I collapsed into bed and cried myself to sleep.

Fortunately, I continued my practice of writing my night-time dreams in a journal. For over 30 years I've recorded my dreams every morning before I get out of bed. (I also write in the middle of the night when I wake from an intense dream. I've learned that I can rarely remember them in the morning.) Sometimes, as my day progresses, I'll even remember a detail and add it to my journal. My dreams have become such an important aspect of my spiritual practice, I frequently turn to them for wisdom and guidance, and at that moment I needed them more than ever. Over those first few weeks I had a series of dreams that culminated in the image of a woman standing in a clearing in the forest, in a circle of light. Her feet were shoulder-width apart in a stance of power, her head tilted back to receive the sun on her face. Her arms were thrust in the air in a show of victory—and—she was single-breasted! My treatment decision was made.

My partner, unconvinced of the legitimacy of my dream, was certain I was over-reacting by choosing mastectomy over my other options. But I knew differently. It was rare that I said "no," and when I did, it was never well received. We were both accustomed to me giving in to keep the peace. This time, it was different. I had a life to save—mine—and if ever there was an appropriate time to behave selfishly, this was it. I surprised us both when I stood firmly in the middle of the living room, hands on my hips, and said, "This is my cancer, and I'll deal with it my way." It was the defining moment of our relationship.

All my life I had been agreeable, trained to be attentive to the needs and desires of those around me. Everyone I cared about—family, friends, partners, co-workers, even my students and congregation—could depend on me. But along the way I had neglected to make my own needs a priority, and it was time for that to change. Over the course of my life I had given myself away in increments that were so small, they appeared negligible in the moment. Finally, these tiny pieces of me had added up and were taking their toll: I was about to give away a body part.

And it didn't escape me that my breast was symbolic of nurturing others—the exact body part that a woman would give away after a life-time of taking care of others ahead of herself. As time went on in my search for an understanding of this dis-ease, it became clear that breast cancer is on the rise in our culture as a wake-up call for women to value themselves at least as much as they value others. Perhaps, when we have all internalized a healthy respect for ourselves, breast cancer will begin to fade.

Gradually I saw that cancer had something valuable to offer—it was time to start saying "yes" to myself. There was a gift in this experience, if only I could manage to stay open enough to receive it. As this awareness began to take hold, the sense of betrayal I had originally felt slowly melted away. Bolstered with the conviction that this disease was a nudge from God intended to help me love myself better, I arrived at the hospital with confidence, ready for my mastectomy. I knew from my dreams that I would be fine—cancer free and stronger than ever. Two days later, leaving the hospital in the obligatory wheelchair, I wore a tiara and pink boa as I waved goodbye to the staff who had cared for me so well. I felt like royalty, reigning over my own life, boldly stepping into my future as a changed woman. There would be no turning back.

When the bandages were removed a week later, I was nervous. Reluctant to glance down as the nurse cut through the layers of gauze, I kept my gaze on the ceiling. She "ooed" and "ahhed," saying what a beautiful job my surgeon had done, but I wanted to be alone the first time I saw my new body. Back at home, in the privacy of my own bathroom, I stood in front of the mirror, closed my eyes, unzipped my sweatshirt and dropped it to the floor. Taking a deep breath, I opened my eyes and looked. The feelings of disfigurement I had expected, were not there. Knowing I could not ask to be cancer free and have a body that was unscarred, I tenderly ran my hand over the flat side of my chest, and smiled. This is what a body, emptied of cancer, looks like. My dreams had prepared me well.

The pathology report was stellar. No lymph node involvement combined with my choice of mastectomy meant no chemo, no radiation, and no Tamoxifen. I felt victorious the day my oncologist uttered the words, "You're cured. Go out and have a good life."

For the next few months I lived in ecstasy. Spring held the promise of new life like never before. I'd lived in the same town for forty years, but everything felt fresh and exhilarating. I was especially thrilled to be alive to watch my son graduate from college. But there was pain developing in my back, growing stronger every day. Although I was content with my one-breasted body, the imbalance of weight was causing my spine to twist, and I succumbed to the need for reconstructive surgery.

The first reconstruction—a reduction of my remaining breast and an implant on the mastectomy side—was unsuccessful. I was overwhelmed and frustrated at the prospect of more surgery; what I really wanted was to be done with it all. It didn't help matters that my partner, angry with the whole situation and unable to accept my decision to have a mastectomy, scheduled an out-of-town business trip during each of my surgeries. We were both deeply affected by this threat on my life, but I felt increasingly abandoned and resentful.

These absences were taking a toll on our relationship, and I began to question whether or not this was a marriage worth saving. Rather than wrangle for control of the situation, I decided to use it as an opportunity for growth, a way to push myself further into the world and see where it would lead. I was determined to learn all the lessons that cancer held for me; the loss of my breast would not be wasted.

I learned to call on friends to supply meals and run errands when I was too weak to fend for myself, and joined The Wellness Community where I found strength in sharing with other cancer patients who were also redefining their lives. Strong women began to come forward in my life to serve as compassionate mentors. They taught me how to how to forgive myself for the many ways I'd given myself away, that "no" is a good word to learn to use, and that "nice" is not always in my best interest. They encouraged me to embrace the concept that it is better to ask for forgiveness than beg for permission, and introduced me to the work of Laurel Thatcher Ulrich, a Pulitzer Prize winner, who said: "Well-behaved women rarely make history."

It was hard work examining the behaviors I'd practiced all my life. But it felt like the process of change had taken on a life of its own, and I was just along for the ride. These women cried with me as I grieved for all the time I'd lost by not believing in myself, and laughed with me as I learned to have a more lighthearted and plucky attitude about life. They gave me unlimited safe space to explore every aspect of my being and express the roller coaster of emotions that passed through me—even the ugly emotions. They are responsible for teaching me to embrace myself for who I truly am, not who everyone else wants me to be.

Living moment-to-moment throughout all the operations, emotional upheaval and physical changes, I had very little perspective on time. Two years and five surgeries had passed since my diagnosis. Only now, with a clean bill of health, successfully reconstructed breasts and a shift in the direction of personal strength, did I have the energy to focus on what was happening around me. The losses in my life were enormous. Along with my breast I had lost a partner, a few friends, and even the comfort of familiarity with myself. The changes that took place over those two years—both internally and externally—were dramatic; I felt like a stranger in my own life. Facing the future alone at age fifty-two was frightening, especially with this new brazen attitude that felt both powerful and awkward. It has taken time to learn how to handle my new self gracefully.

Several months after my last surgery, while I was still at home recovering, my friend Maggie went to the Susan G. Komen Walk for the Cure in San Francisco. The ABC-TV booth at the event was staffed by Fran Zone, an executive and communications coach in San Francisco. Fran was offering her expertise, for free, to a survivor who was ready to thrive; a woman who wanted to take her post-cancer life to an entirely new level. Maggie, who had supported and encouraged me over the past two years, signed me up as a candidate. Fran interviewed me by phone the following week, and took me on as her client.

My work is all about empowering women and children, creating healing opportunities in our world. During the last six months of my cancer journey I began having dreams (much the same way that I dreamt of the one-breasted woman in the forest) of working with women and children in Africa. Fran made it her mission to bring my project to life. She put me on the local ABC-TV affiliate to speak about my cancer experience, made a generous personal donation for my travel to Africa, and hosted a fund-raising party to complete my project's financing. I met Fran in September, 2007, and left alone for South Africa in January, 2008 to work with rural Zulu children. All because I allowed myself to stay open to the multitude of changes that entered my life along with cancer.

I won't lie; cancer was a challenging struggle. There were many times I wanted to run away and give up. My fears around allowing myself to become someone new and end my ten-year relationship, felt overwhelming. None of it was easy. But now, nearly five years after my diagnosis, I feel like such a winner. Yes, I lost a lot, but what I've gained is even more remarkable: my authentic voice, trust in my intuition, respect for my value as a woman walking through this world, and the ability to meet my own needs. I still enjoy caring for the loved ones in my life, but I no longer do it at my own expense.

My life has been full since I returned home from Africa: I accepted a position as a hospital chaplain in my home town while I sorted out my divorce; I enjoyed dancing with my son at his wedding last summer; and last fall, fulfilling a long-time yearning in my heart, I relocated to northern New Mexico. I was pretty certain life couldn't get any better. But on Mother's Day this year, much to my delight, I received sonogram photos announcing my first grandchild!

All my life I've wanted to feel whole and content, comfortable in my own skin, excited about life, and confident of my place in the world. Maybe my own thoughts did attract breast cancer to me, because that disease—such an unexpected vehicle of transformation—has provided exactly what I asked for: a deep knowing that I am whole and good, just the way I am!

In the beginning I hated that I had to go through cancer. Now, I wouldn't give back the experience for all the world. And me and God? We're fine. God is growing accustomed to me living this unrestricted life. Actually, I think that might have been Her plan all along!

# 3.

# Ain't Got Time To Die!

## BY BRENDA BEST

*Brenda Best was born and raised in the horse country of Virginia, where she trained and rode horses professionally. She is a U.S. Navy Veteran and has been an elementary educator since 1989. Brenda was diagnosed in 2008 with breast cancer and is now beginning her third year of thriving. She lives in San Diego, California, with her daughter and mini-zoo of supportive pets. Brenda can be contacted at best.brenda@att.net.*

*The untold want, by life and land ne'er granted,*
*Now, Voyager, sail thou forth, to seek and find.*
*- Walt Whitman, The Untold Want*

Everyone counts on warranties and insurance policies, don't they? What about you? Would you even consider buying a car or a washing machine or a stove without a warranty? Of course not! Well, I knew that there was no guarantee I would never get cancer, but the checks I wrote to support cancer research and the Susan G. Komen 3-Day for the Cure somehow provided me with a false sense of security. Surely this generosity would be my insurance policy against getting breast cancer.

When I was first diagnosed with breast cancer, I was embarrassed. How in the world had I allowed this to happen to me? Weren't the checks big enough? Should I have covered my bases with even greater generosity?

I knew, of course, that such questions made absolutely no sense. Looking for valid explanations was futile. This was simply a journey that I would have to make. I was not going to allow myself to die! No way, I had too much stuff to do, things to accomplish! I did not have time to die! I wanted to be here to see my daughter graduate, to see her marry. My grandbabies had to know what a great "Nanny" I was going to be! This heinous disease was NOT going to take that away from me!

With my diagnosis, I became as a wanderer. I imagined myself a Bedouin roaming the arid deserts. I felt lost and alone, in spite of all the loving support my family and friends gave me. This trip I was on didn't seem to have a lick of logic to it. I had no idea where I would be going or whom I would meet along the way. But I did know that I must travel great distances and could take with me only what I could carry. Pack light. Now that was always a motto I could live with.

And so it began. I researched. I read. I pondered. I prayed, and oh yes, I tried to bargain.

Yet, despite the tide of support from family, friends and my medical team, who swept me from diagnosis through treatment and surgeries, I was still that Bedouin wanderer. Persistently searching for the perfect oasis, scared to death that it would be unattainable. Now that is where my journey truly began. Little did I know that this was the moment I was beginning the metamorphosis from survivor to thriver.

So what is the true line drawn in the dirt that separates surviving and thriving? For me it was when I transitioned from the nuts and bolts of merely getting through each day to truly and absolutely living each day to the fullest. I was a survivor when it was all about me simply making it through each day, putting one foot in front of the other - faking it until I made it. I became a thriver when I began to give back all the gifts I had received. That happened as I began to synergize my energy with the energy and vitality of my friends and family and all the other thrivers in the world. Revitalizing myself by means of making the most of every minute in every hour. My oasis was about to become visible on the horizon.

I had gone into a lovely little shop for cancer patients and survivors, determined to find the perfect breasts. Well, why not? Now I had the opportunity that very few women possess. I could decide upon the ideal size and shape! And why not have several sets? You know, different-sized breast prosthetics for different occasions? Unfortunately, once inside the store I soon found myself sickeningly ill at ease. I was not ready for this part of my journey. Quickly I turned to leave, when a wonderfully intuitive woman handed me a copy of Breast Cancer Wellness Magazine. Smiling broadly she said, "Here, take this, you might find it interesting." So as to hush her up quickly and not detain my departure, I grabbed the magazine and hurried out the door. Little did I know that this magazine would turn out to be my exact deliverance!

I literally jumped into the car, and my daughter who was waiting there for me, asked, "Are you all right?"

"Yes, why do you ask?" I snapped.

"Because you look like you saw a ghost."

"Just not ready for this part, yet" was my reply.

Later, at home, flipping through the magazine, I read wonderful stories of breast cancer survivors. They were successful and healthy women. I was amazed and uplifted. These women were celebrating their lives - not simply surviving, but THRIVING! They were going on trips, living life and having fun. I wanted that! At that very moment I resolved to go on the next cruise. These ladies had something I wanted. Are you beginning to see that oasis? Well, I was.

That Breast Cancer Thrivers cruise was the best thing I have ever done for myself. I realized that I was not the lonely Bedouin. There existed a whole gaggle of us! We just had to find one another. Together we helped each other along on our journey toward our oasis. We laughed together, we cried together, we shared our experiences and frustrations. We shared our fears, hopes and loves. And, yes, we do have a big wonderful oasis out there! Filled with beautiful women who are breast cancer thrivers.

Since my first cruise with the BCT group, I have been networking with the most incredible and supportive group of thriving women in the universe! I have made strong and close friendships for life. We live all over the world, but we share a common bond. No, not cancer, my friend. The common bond we share is—we are THRIVERS!

My surgeon calls us the largest sorority on earth. You know, I think he has that right! No matter how you look at it, life is short. Every moment needs to be cherished. I plan to live hard, love incessantly and come flying in to the end of it all by the seat of my pants with a big "Wahoo!" I wouldn't have missed this trip for anything!

*Dedicated to my daugher Michaella, whose "old soul" wisdom sustained and lifted me along this journey.*

# 4.

# My Journey From Incurable to Incredible

## BY TAMI BOEHMER

*Tami Boehmer lives with her husband Mike, daughter Chrissy and furry feline AJ in Cincinnati, Ohio. After being diagnosed with a metastatic breast cancer recurrence, Tami began interviewing survivors nationwide who survived and thrived years beyond what medical science predicted. Tami compiled these inspirational stories into her book, From Incurable to Incredible: Cancer Survivors Who Beat the Odds. You can learn more about her book, as well as valuable information on healing the body, mind and spirit; on her Web site and blog www.miraclesurvivors.com.*

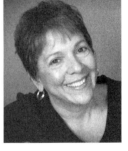

Staring at my breast surgeon's forlorn face that February afternoon in 2008, I knew something was terribly wrong.

I'd insisted on seeing her a month earlier than my regular check-up because of a large lump I discovered in my right armpit. I had worried from time to time about some swelling and hardness. Since the swelling would go down, my surgeon thought it was probably hormonal. I was so relieved, I didn't question it.

Now I wanted answers. My worst nightmare came true – a recurrence. Even worse, this time it was stage IV breast cancer. An oncologist from a very prestigious institution told me, "You could live two years or twenty years, but you will die of breast cancer."

I felt devastated, and then I got angry. Who is she tell me how long I had to live? I had an eight-year-old daughter and a wonderful husband to love. I wasn't going anywhere!

After I "beat" cancer the first time more than five years previously, I promised myself that if it ever returned, I would fight it with everything I had. That's the way I always react to crisis situations. I spring into action.

I realized I needed to talk with other cancer survivors who didn't accept doctors' predictions... people who beat the odds. And I was determined to find out how they did it so I could do it myself.

I thought of Buzz Sheffield, a volunteer prayer chaplain at our church. Buzz was always up in the front row with a snazzy suit and dazzling smile. You could almost see the light of God emanating from him.

I remembered a year previously seeing Buzz sitting in the courtyard of the large, teaching hospital where I worked. It was a beautiful sunny day, and Buzz looked peaceful as he read a book. As usual, I was in a rush. As an ambitious public relations specialist, I was dashing to meet a TV reporter who was doing a story on one of our patients.

He told me he was waiting for tests, and the last ones showed he had cancer all over his body. I stood there in shock. I would have never guessed that this active, robust man had anything wrong with him. We didn't know each other well at the time, but I felt a special connection with him from that moment on.

After church that Sunday, I asked him about his tests and his illness. He told me he had carcinoid cancer, a rare, slow-moving disease that often attacks the intestines and other parts of the body where hormones are produced. Four years earlier, doctors told him he had three to six months to live. His cancer was so extensive, chemotherapy wasn't an option. He refused to listen to their doomsday predictions and chose to focus on healing through prayer, giving back to others, and healthy nutrition and exercise. To look at him and his active lifestyle, I knew whatever he is doing was working.

The first night after getting my dreaded diagnosis, I needed to talk to someone who understood what I was going through, and most important, was doing well. I gave Buzz a call.

"Tell me everything you are doing," I said, anxious to emulate him. "I'm taking notes."

The first thing he told me was to not give up, stay in the moment, and remain positive. He also told me about his strong spiritual connection, healthy diet and exercise routine. I started following his advice as I went through ten months of chemotherapy treatments.

I started making significant changes in my lifestyle. I left my stressful job and made exercise, prayer, visualization, and affirmations a daily routine. I abandoned my chronic sugar addiction and switched to a healthy, whole-foods diet. I focused on serving others in my breast cancer support group, at church and by delivering meals to elderly people in my neighborhood. Most of all, I began to devote time to enriching all of my relationships, especially with my family, myself and God.

Remarkably, my side effects were minimal and my tumors shrank with every scan. But still, I fought off depression and was haunted by the sinking feeling I was going to die. With all the focus on myself and getting well, I felt useless and empty. I was searching for meaning in my life.

My husband and I work in public relations and always dreamed of writing a book together. In June, three months into my chemo treatments, we went on vacation with Mike's family to a beautiful lake in Canada. On one of my daily morning walks, an idea popped into my mind. "Why not write a book about other advanced stage cancer patients and how they beat the odds?" I thought it would be therapeutic for me and, more important, help others. I soon began interviewing cancer survivors from around the country for my book, *From Incurable to Incredible*.

Finally, at the end of my treatments, I heard those three little words every girl (with cancer) dreams about: "You're in remission." Cancer returned since then, but I know it will just be a matter of time before I hear these words again.

For me, cancer was a wake-up call. If I didn't learn the first time around, this second bout with cancer certainly caught my attention. Cancer has brought many blessings that I would not have realized without this daunting challenge. Writing my book is certainly one of them. The process of interviewing the amazing individuals featured in the book and writing their stories has been extremely therapeutic to me. I include their stories, along with ways to heal the body, mind and spirit in my blog called Miracle Survivors.

Here are a few lessons I learned along my cancer journey:

## Find good mentors

Several years before my recurrence, a man named Terry McBride came to our church to speak. Terry, after countless surgeries and years of self-healing, had overcome a dire e-coli infection in his spine that doctors predicted would leave him paralyzed. Terry never gave up, and today he is free from disease with no physical impairments.

My husband Mike and I both read Terry's book, *The Hell I Can't*. We heard he was "coaching" a member of our church over the phone. Mike e-mailed Terry and asked if he had any ideas for our situation. He told us he had plenty of ideas and told us to contact him.

So, every Wednesday, I talked with Terry. He suggested a daily routine of visualization, prayer and affirmations and taught me how to guide my body to heal. He was the one who convinced me, in his "football-coach, no-nonsense way," to not return to my grueling and stressful job.

Terry showed me that I had the power to create—with God—healing and anything else I wanted. I learned how to transform fear and self doubt into faith in myself and my divinity. He gave me hope.

## Listen to children

My greatest teacher was and continues to be my daughter, Chrissy. Being a person who worked all my life, I was feeling guilty for taking medical leave from work and focusing so much on self care. I even began to wonder if my life held any meaning.

Chrissy often told me that cancer was one of the best things to happen because it allowed us to get closer and spend more time together. One night when I was putting Chrissy to bed, she looked in my eyes and said, "You are setting a good example for me because you're being so spiritual and taking care of yourself."

Yet she noted that I needed to maintain some balance. Noticing me reading yet another spiritual book, she encouraged me to stop taking myself so seriously. "Sometimes being spiritual means taking a break. Relax and have fun, Mommy."

I was worried that we might be scaring Chrissy by being so open about the cancer, but that was far from the truth. By taking care of myself and focusing on spirituality, she was learning a valuable lesson.

## Flex your spiritual muscles

Many times I would feel alone, although I knew I had so many people in my life who cared about me. Fears and self-doubt came up, then I would beat myself up for not being positive. My bi-monthly scans would bring up emotion, too. My head was filled with anxious thoughts, "How do I live with this uncertainty? What if, what if, what if..."

To combat this, I had a daily routine of taking, what I called, "walks with God." I find that nature brings me closer to a higher power that creates all living things. While I was enjoying the beautiful breeze and sunshine, God and I would have a little talk. I would ask God for guidance and to show me how to heal my life. Soon, a sense of peace washed over me. I felt the knot in my stomach unwind and chest relax.

I began to build my faith that God will fulfill my heart's desire. God did not bring me this far to let me down.

## Empower yourself with daily rituals

I knew I needed to do the footwork and not leave it all up to God. So, I carried my toolkit with me at all times. This included books, DVDs, affirmations, even a picture I drew of my white blood cells attacking cancer cells.

While I was waiting in the car to pick up my daughter Chrissy from school or in line at the store, I would visualize my immune system melting the cancer cells away. As I drank water—and lots of it—I would see myself cleansing the residue of dead cancer cells out of my body. While taking a shower, I talked to my body, urging it to clear out the cancer and thanking it for its amazing work.

To see how I could build my immune system, I consulted with a naturopath physician and read the books, *Beating Cancer with Nutrition* by Patrick Quillin and *Anticancer: A New Way of Life* by David Servan Schreiber, MD. I spent time purchasing organic produce and supplements with cancer-fighting properties. I even gave up sugar, which I loved, with the exception of really dark chocolate. I started using eco-friendly cleaners and natural shampoos and lotions.

All of these practices gave me a sense of power; that I was doing something concrete to support my healing. And it seemed to be working. My side effects were minimal from chemotherapy, and each scan showed the cancer was shrinking.

## Attitude really does impact health

I realize, that left to its own devices, my mind can automatically go to the negative, worried mode. As I continued to do affirmations, it became more natural for these positive thoughts to replace the negative ones.

At the same time, I learned that it is not healthy to try to be positive all the time. Tears and expressions of anger can be cleansing, as long as I don't hold on to them. It takes more energy to suppress these feelings than to express them.

## You are more than a disease

Sometimes I could get so caught up with fighting cancer, I started to identify it as part of me. I would also notice it in others when I went to cancer support groups and sometimes in the chemo suite.

I had cancer. It did not have me. I would repeat these words like a mantra: "I am not a disease or treatments. It is something that I am experiencing right now, but it is not my identity. It is a temporary bump in the road—the scary part of my story—but it will pass. I can create a happy ending."

## Be grateful

One thing I know is that I really need to appreciate every day and those people around me. I also learned that it was just as important to express gratitude to God and others as it was to feel it. By being grateful for all things, even the challenges, I brought more good into my life. This experience has shown me that I cannot take life for granted.

# 5.

# I Finally Truly Feel Beautiful

## BY KATRINA BOS

*Four years after losing her mother to breast cancer, Katrina Bos found lumps growing in one of her breasts. Through the guidance of a wise man, Katrina chose an alternative way through her illness and experienced a miraculous healing which altered her life forever. This story and the subsequent research findings became the subject of her book, "What if you could skip the Cancer?" which was published in 2009. Her experience led her to restore a historic train station (www.eaststreetstation.ca ) where she helps others to see what's going on inside of them so they can heal and move forward. She can be reached at katrina@eaststreetstation.ca. www.katrinabos.com.*

beau-ty *[byoo-te]*

1. the quality present in a thing or person that gives intense pleasure or deep satisfaction to the mind, whether arising from sensory manifestations (as shape, color, sound, etc.), a meaningful design or pattern, or something else (as a personality in which high spiritual qualities are manifest).
2. an individually pleasing or beautiful quality; grace; charm

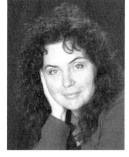

I never thought of myself as beautiful. As a child, I didn't worry about what I looked like. When I became a teenager, I definitely cared—and I had acne, tiny little breasts and kinky hair. I had none of the "look" that you had to have to be considered beautiful.

So, I worked hard to "become beautiful". I bought the right clothes. I tried to make my hair go right (which at the time was getting it to feather back like Farrah Fawcett's). I used acne medication and lots of makeup. But it didn't work. All the "right" people didn't pay me any more attention. I wasn't any more beautiful. I was just the same homely kid with lots of make-up and hairspray. University was a little better. The idea of what was beautiful seemed to be broader. More different styles were accepted. But I could always find other women who were more beautiful, thinner, and better than me. At that point in my life, I was sure that this lack of real beauty would stand in the way of me ever finding a man who would love me—which was really depressing.

But then I found one. Not only did he think I was beautiful, he actually loved me. Not only did he love me, he wanted to marry me. Wow!!! You'd think that this would be enough for me to finally accept that perhaps I was beautiful. Perhaps I was worth loving. Perhaps I was actually alright.

Alas, it wasn't so. As the years went on, when my husband told me that I was beautiful and that he loved me, I was sure that he just wanted to get lucky (which might have been true—but it didn't have to take away from the fact that he DID think that I was beautiful).

It wasn't until a few years later when I was faced with lumps growing in my breasts that things really started to change for me from the inside out. We had been married for six years. I had a four year-old son and a two-year-old daughter.

My mom had died of breast cancer 4 years earlier. Her sister had died of cancer 20 years earlier. My grandmother had died because of cancer when my mom was 14. So, cancer was definitely the "big bad" that would help me to stop and really look at my life and make some serious changes.

One thing that I really had to look at was the fact that I really wasn't living the life I was meant to live. Sure, I was doing everything "right". I married a good man, had babies, made jam, cleaned the house, and even chaired the parents' council. Plus, we had a dairy farm. So between household chores and the needs of my babies, there were cows to milk and farm work to be done. The needs were endless. And the days pretty much ran together.

No matter how upbeat I tried to be, the reality was that I was depressed. Sure, I could always see the silver lining. Sure, I could make the best of any situation. In fact, on top of everything that I needed to do, I could even help anyone else who needed something.

The fact that I was actually depressed was a real shocker for me. As far as I was concerned, I was upbeat. I was the person who depressed people came to for help. There wasn't any way that I was depressed. I mean, compared to whom? And if I was depressed, what was I depressed about?

The reality was that I had spent my whole life burying who I really was trying to become someone else—someone who other people would like, would respect, would think was a beautiful person. If I had ideas or thoughts that weren't acceptable or that would cause too big a wave, they were squashed. If my feelings about something might cause someone else discomfort or difficulty, I swallowed them hoping that they'd just disappear. But they didn't. They just festered for decades.

This is one of the great things about facing our own mortality. When we find ourselves wondering if we are going to live or die, we often start looking at our lives differently. We wonder why we aren't being honest with ourselves. We wonder what we are waiting for. We wonder why we aren't doing the things that we really want to be doing.

And so, I started listening to that still, small voice inside that I had been ignoring for most of my life. At first, the challenge was simply sorting out all the "voices" in my head. Which one was my own inner voice? Then, I started to act on what I heard. Most often, it was small things. Sometimes it was just being honest with someone about whether I wanted to do something or not. Sometimes it was choosing to take dance lessons. But most of the time it was just giving an honest "yes" or "no" answer to any question posed.

As time went on, I was able to listen to bigger inner thoughts. Once, I realized that I really wanted to open a dance studio with my dance instructor—and I actually did. Later, I realized that I loved to write and "my little voice" said that it would be great to be a regular columnist in the local paper. I wrote some sample articles, presented them to the publisher and voila, I had my own column. What was really wonderful was that as my life started to become what I was actually about, I started to really love myself. Bit by bit, I started liking who I was. I was really enjoying life for the first time in a long time. And the coolest thing was that it was truly MY life—totally based on my inner design.

Today, people often tell me that I "sparkle". That really interests me. Over a 20 year span, I went from "frumpy and depressed" to "sparkly". And the core thing that I changed was that my outsides now reflect my insides.

I am no thinner. My hair is the same as it's been for 30 years. My skin is no different and my wardrobe hasn't changed. But I am truly happy. I really love my life.

My life is a true reflection of who I actually am—and I finally, truly feel beautiful.

# 6.

# Arranging the Letters, Arranging My Life

## BY MARY CARWILE

*Mary Catherine Carwile walked to the edge of her fears and took a leap of faith. Twice divorced and just after her youngest son graduated high school, there was yet another test. This time it was breast cancer. A year after the surgeries and clean bill of health, Mary took another leap. She accepted a dare from a friend and became a flight attendant, despite her fear of flying. Mary is the award winning author of Heartstrings at 35,000 Feet, True Stories That Will Melt Your Heart and Heartstrings and Pink Ribbons, Finding Comfort Until There's a Cure. She is an inspiration/motivational speaker. www.MaryCarwile.com*

I've always liked English. In high school I loved the way the words snaked over the page as I diagramed a sentence; was fascinated to find that words could change my mood, my attitude, my outlook on life; found that words to a song could completely undo me or take me to a place of calm or happiness. Words. Try changing a letter or two. Even one letter can change its entire meaning. Take "better" and "bitter." Just one letter separates being more proficient at something or becoming an angry person.

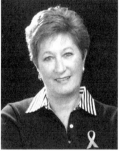

"Survive." "Thrive." The two words end the same and sound very similar, don't they? Their meanings, however, are nothing alike.

Being raised in a small, conservative Midwestern town, we weren't typically risk takers. I learned at an early age to be very careful in life; to not do anything that would put me at risk. It was important to fit in; to make sure the neighbors wouldn't talk. We were surviving. We learned if life dealt us a hard blow, we just tried to survive and tough it out. As I got a bit older and married, those unspoken "rules" began unraveling.

I started listening to motivational tapes, going to motivational speakers and reading positive books in my early twenties. I loved the enthusiasm and energy this brought to my life. I tried to take on the "glass is half full" approach to life. I had all that knowledge in my head and I loved it.

Then I was tested. The universe wanted to see if I could move that knowledge from my head... to my heart.

When my husband of nearly fourteen years came home one night to tell me he wanted a divorce, my world was turned up-side-down. I remember being too stunned to even cry. Eventually I began recalling what I'd earlier learned. I remembered what I'd been reading, hearing.

As the groundwork had been laid, the change I felt was small at first. It was only a tiny, quiet voice whispering, Mary, you have no choice. You have to do this!

"Well," I said back to myself, "I do have a choice." I had a challenge ahead of me—a big challenge. I had a six year old son and was just six weeks away from having my second son. The children needed me. Something registered inside me, something I'd heard in a sermon sometime before. "You can choose to be better or bitter," it said. Those words kept repeating in my head... better or bitter, better or bitter, better or bitter. Right then and there, I made a conscious choice. I had to be strong before I could be a good mother to my boys. Surprising even to me, the very thing I was most afraid of—raising my children alone—was the challenge that made me find my own strength.

I was by then living in a small, ski resort village in Colorado. I began to thrive. I had examples all around me of people thriving in life. I witnessed people skiing with only one leg; winters that seemed, at times, to just run together; people that had chosen where they wanted to live, what they wanted to do, how they would enjoy life. The feeling was conagious. I began to take more risks, challenge my ideas. I began my own business. I came to realize that the feeling of being uncomfortable was actually a good thing. It meant I was growing, changing, thriving.

Nearly twenty years after I'd first felt those twinges of strength, just after my youngest son had graduated high school and left home, I was tested once again.

Waiting in the small room in just my paper gown, I was surprised to see the doctor coming in behind my mammography technician. This can't be good news, I remember thinking. He told me they'd "found something" on my mammogram, that I'd need a biopsy and "don't worry," he added. I chose to believe him and went about my day without worry. Worrying never helps anyway, does it?

After my biopsy, I waited several days to hear from my doctor. When she finally reached me, it was nearly eleven PM. I'd been trying to keep my mind occupied and had been typing on my laptop when I finally decided she wasn't going to call that night. Just as I logged off my computer, my phone rang. You see, that was nearly eleven years ago. My laptop was plugged into my phone line.

At that late hour and in my heightened state, my doctor gave me five words that changed my life forever, "Mary, you have breast cancer."

Once again, only this time much faster, I found that place inside myself; that place where I knew I needed to be strong, to deal and move on. That's how I looked at life. It was a bump in my road, for sure, but it wasn't going to stop me, whatever the outcome.

I had to wait nearly a month before there was a surgery time for me. During that time, I found my strength growing. I was scared, to be sure, but now I was becoming a part of this. I had choices to make. I surely hadn't consciously chosen breast cancer but I most certainly did have a choice in how I was going to react to having breast cancer.

I remember late one night, driving over the high mountain pass to reach my home from the city. As I drove alone through the dark, I listened to a tape by Dr. Bernie Siegel. He said something on that tape that brought me full circle; gave me just what I needed to be much more than a breast cancer survivor. Dr. Siegel was telling his listeners... me... that he had one especially wonderful woman he was seeing that was going through breast cancer. She was also going through a divorce. I, too, had just separated from my second husband.

Great timing, don't you think?

The woman Dr. Siegel talked about had a mantra. "I'm getting rid of a boob and an ass all at the same time." I laughed when I heard it but it rang totally true for me. You see, I believe that I got breast cancer because I stuffed all of my feelings during my unhappy marriage. I'd always smiled and said, "Oh, I'm fine" whenever someone asked about me/ my life. I never let on how miserable I was. Her mantra became my mantra. I visualized all the junk in my life sitting right there in my right breast.

As I was wheeled into surgery a couple of weeks later, the mantra was running through my head. "I'm getting rid of a boob and an ass all at the same time," I repeated in my head as I fell into a deep sleep. I knew, with certainty, that all the junk in my life was being removed right along with my breast tissue. I would wake up with neither my breast cancer nor all the messy divorce stuff anymore. I knew it then; I feel it now.

My life has moved in an upward direction then. I moved from my mountain home to the city, accepted a new and challenging job as a flight attendant (in my mid-fifties, with a fear of flying), met (on a plane) and married a wonderful man, wrote two books and am now thrilled to be sharing my story with other women in my talk, "Soaring Above the Turbulence."

It's amazing to me. Changing my attitude... and just a few letters in a word... and I went form being a survivor to a thriver. It's made all the difference in the world.

BreastCancerWellness.org

# 7.

# Thrive in Five

## BY JANET CHAMBERS

*Janet resides in Northern Kentucky with her husband, Mike. She has 3 daughters, and a stepson that have blessed her with 8 grandchildren. She is an eleven year breast cancer survivor. In 2002, she founded I Have Wings Breast Cancer Foundation (www.ihavewings.org) and is currently the Executive Director. The loves of her life: Her husband, the foundation, her children and grandchildren, her flower garden, and her Brittney Spaniel bless most of her time and energy!*

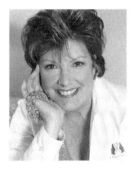

The year of 1993 started with a BANG! My life as I knew it seemed to be falling apart around me like a clown car at the circus! My marriage of fifteen years was failing, I had three adorable daughters who needed stability, and I needed a car and a better job. Like many daughters, I fell back on my own mother and in March, 1993, myself, and my three daughters Linda, Shelly and Kelsey moved in with her.

One night after dinner, mom said "Honey, you just need to get back to your roots! Let's go to church tonight. They're having a congregational healing mass and you just can't do this pain alone anymore!"

In an effort to please mom and, after all, I did just turn her quiet lifestyle into chaos, I replied "Fine". 7 p.m. church was packed. Forgiveness must be in high demand these days, or maybe it just seemed that way to me. So I prayed.

"Dear God, you know I have not always lived according to your word. I certainly have not made the best choices or honored Your will. Please love me anyway. Send Your spirit to heal my insecurities that keep You from entering my life. Forgive me of anything I've done consciously or unconsciously that pushed You out of my life. Oh, and thank you ahead of time for hearing my prayers. Amen."

With mom happy and that behind me, I was feeling forgiven and recharged to get on with my life. I felt invincible. Now I was ready to conquer anything in my path- or was I?

Time just seemed to fly by while living with mom. We enjoyed a cup of tea at night while watching updates on the OJ trial. A year and a half later (August 1994), I bought a small 2 bedroom house not far from mom, convenient for the girls to get off the bus and walk to our home later. I even started line dancing and going out with friends again. Two years later (June 1996), after being courted by Mike, got married in Saint Thomas and upon return threw a reception with our now 'Brady Bunch' family. In 1997, we brought our dream home and 1998 ushered in a new job that I really loved. I thought life was good and that

God must have heard my prayer. This brings us up to 1999, just after my 40th birthday. July 3, 1999. Ringing phone cuts the morning silence. I answer with a sleepy "Hello". "Janet?... I'm sorry, but I wanted to let you know as soon as possible that your biopsy results are back (silence): It's breast cancer."

I think at that point I defined the term "uncontrollable crying". A lot had happened since 1993. God, did you really hear my prayer? Had my day to day been so busy that I forgot to pray? Was I so consumed in my new life and raising my children that I unconsciously ignored the most important aspect of it? Then those five little words mom so desperately pleaded with me to absorb, came back... "Go back to your roots".

With the help of the scripture in my Jerusalem Bible, I soon found out my personal, practical, secrets of a THRIVER. THRIVE in FIVE!

## 1. REST

*Matthew 11: 28-30*
*Come to me, all of you who labor and are overburdened, and I will give you rest.*

I think I mentioned that Mike and I purchased a new home. Shortly after moving in, we started to purge an area of the backyard of annoying, never tended weeds that were climbing our trees. Similar to cancer, the weeds were out of control, destructive and ultimately suffocating the life right out of the once healthy trees. After I was diagnosed, Mike finished the project by creating a healing garden. A place of solace where I could restore my energy, renew my spirit, meditate or pray, grieve or just have a good cry (as we all need a good cry once in awhile when going through chemo). The garden was at the back of the yard, which for some, was just a skip but for me, Miss No Energy, seemed like an all day hike! It turned out to be an excellent place to escape reality, if even for a few minutes. Not many of us get our eight hours at night (especially if you're waking yourself up in the middle of the night, munching on dry cereal to prevent nausea), so an occasional siesta in the garden was just what I needed.

## 2. REMOVE THE GARBAGE

*Philippians 4: 8*
*Fill your minds with everything that is true, everything that is noble, everything that is good and pure, everything that we love and honor and everything that can be thought virtuous or worthy of praise.*

*Psalm 90: 14*
*Let us wake in the morning filled with your love and sing and be happy all our days.*

Remember when you were reading your favorite comic book or magazine and your mom said to you "Stop reading that junk, garbage in, garbage out"! I think its way broader than that now! Garbage enters our lives so quickly, on so many levels, that sometimes it just sneaks in without us giving it a thought. Preservatives in our foods, electronic games,

TV's, computers, cell phones, pornography, twitter, facebook. Everything is accessible at our fingertips and in a moment's notice, life is getting faster and more furious! After stumbling across this insightful passage in Philippians, I religiously made "Me Time" each morning and immediately added more organic fresh fruit and vegetables into my diet. You wouldn't start exercising without a warm up. Why start you day without a mental warm up? This is a practice I continue today. Usually, I enjoy my morning coffee and my Bible on the deck outside the kitchen. I thought it was so quiet and peaceful until one day a friend said "Janet, where are you? It sounds like you're in paradise!" I laughed! I guess it was paradise! My little paradise of robins singing, bees buzzing, hummingbirds zipping, woodpeckers knocking, locusts playing out a live concert and doves cooing. My very loud, peaceful paradise! Where is your peaceful paradise? THRIVERS learn quickly to remove the garbage!

## 3. PUT ON A NEW DRESS

*Ephesians 4:22-24*
*You must give up your old way of life; you must put aside your old self, which gets corrupted by following illusory desires. Your mind must be renewed by a spiritual revolution, so that you can put on a new self that has been created in God's way, in the goodness and holiness of the truth.*

Have you ever put on an outfit and started to head for the door, just to turn around and change to a completely different dress? Yes, I am not proud to admit it, but I have too! I learned that to THRIVE through cancer sometimes we need a change of surroundings; I call it "putting on a new dress" or as the Bible says "put on a new self" if you prefer! We need to get out of our hum drum routines once and awhile, remove ourselves from unhealthy situations or a negative atmosphere in order to heal. Out with the old, in with the new! A change in venue, so to speak for our mind, body and soul! You can start with small changes as I did or to a whole lifestyle revolution. Mine started the nights before chemo treatments. We were a two income family, with 4 children in private schools. There was no time for me to be sick or take a leave of absence. So, I savored my energy for the work week. My boss was great and I frequently took work home, but I couldn't take advantage. So, each night I ate a quick snack and headed to bed, totally and utterly exhausted. Every night EXCEPT the nights before chemo. Those nights called for a long bubble bath, soft music, a cup of herbal tea and a book. Sometimes I fell asleep in the tub! Something different, something relaxing, something that said; "By golly, tonight I'm something special!"

Since cancer, my lifestyle has had a serious makeover. I realize that I AM something special, EVERYDAY! Things that seem to hold great importance before cancer seem mundane now. Removing negativity, changing old habits into new positive experiences is the new norm.

Now I'm sure you can make a ton of significant life fulfilling changes and the Good Book isn't referencing a bubble bath, but hey, we all need to start someplace!! Changing one routine could change another, and another. Before you know it, you have replaced several bad habits with good ones! Tada! Welcome the new you!

## 4. REJOICE: FIND LAUGHTER AND MAKE SOMEONE LAUGH

*Colossians 3:16-17*
*With gratitude in your hearts, sing psalms and hymns and inspired songs to God*

*Psalm 47: 1*
*Clap your hands, all you peoples, acclaim God with shouts of joy*

Be glad, express joy, sing, laugh! It really is healing! I could share a bazillion funny stories about my cancer journey. Like the night of our Halloween bonfire. Unfortunately for me, I naturally inherited the "vain" gene from my mom. Someone told her in high school that if she cut her eyelashes off, they would come back twice as thick. You guessed it, they didn't, and she spent her entire life utilizing her children to put her false lashes meticulously on, one at a time. I was, of course, the best at putting them on, so I frequently got the privilege of helping her. Being so experienced, you understand, I just had to wear false eyelashes after mine fell out! Unfortunately for me, I must have gotten just a little too close to the fire! However, it was a perfect night to have the funniest, scariest, most twisted and snarly eyelashes. What a hoot and what a super disguise!

But one of the funniest was the night the new boy came over. My oldest daughter Linda, was a teenager and one of her high school goals was to attend every other local high school's prom. Which means we should have installed a revolving door for the new boys every week! One evening during a rather quiet Friday dinner, I decided not to put on my wig or scarf. Loud chiming of the door bell broke our line of conversation. Sternly, I looked around the table and said "Okay, which one of you invited someone over?" All heads were shaking no... Linda jumped to answer the door. As she lets in the newest boy who came courting, she stops him dead in the entry hall and says "You can't go in there, stay right here" stretching out both arms to try to 'hold him captive' in the entry. In a panic, with no scarf, no wig, and no hat I ran into the bathroom, slamming the door! Kelsey, the youngest, exclaims "No worry mom, I'll take care of it!" Kelsey flies upstairs, grabs my wig, and lugs it down the steps... clutching it and swinging it right in front of the "new boy" detained in the entry, and yelling "I got it, I got it"! We never saw him again!

## 5. HOPE

*Isaiah 40: 31*
*But those who hope in the Lord will renew their strength, they will soar on eagles wings; they will run and not grow weary, walk and not be faint.*

My ultimate favorite scripture reading! How powerful, how inspiring, how refreshing are these words! I can't think of anything better... no exhaustion, renewed strength, and no boundaries! When we really have hope, there is no stopping us. Not in life, not in recovery, not in anything! Reading these words inspire me every day to help others soar. After recovery and getting actively involved with cancer survivors in our local community, I Have Wings Breast Cancer Foundation took flight in 2002. WINGS is an acronym for

"With Inspiration No-one Goes Solo". Our mission is the 3 E's: Educate our community on breast cancer prevention. Ease stress of families undergoing a breast cancer diagnosis. And Endorsing breast cancer research. We accomplish this by assisting families emotionally and financially during a cancer diagnosis and supporting Wood Hudson Cancer Research Laboratory. We are located in Northern Kentucky and assist families in the Cincinnati, OH Tri-State area. For more information, go to www.ihavewings.org.

Looking back, Mom was right, I couldn't do it alone and I needed to get back to my roots. I needed some serious change in my life. Whether it's the food we eat, the company we keep, the books we read, or how we accept ourselves. I realize now that God did hear my prayer. That pain prepares you for joy, disease prepares you for health, and that He sent me everything I needed to turn all those difficulties into victories. It's called healing.

Thrive in Five is about turning those negative matters in our lives to positive healing ones... rest, remove the garbage, put on a new dress, laugh and make others laugh, and finally, HOPE!

What are you waiting for? Join me as a THRIVER! There's room in this club for all of us!

BreastCancerWellness.org

# 8.

# What a Journey—from survivor to *Survivor—and,* from survivor to Thriver!

## BY SONJA CHRISTOPHER

*In 2000, Sonja was thrust into the national limelight when, in putting her life back together after diagnosis and treatment for breast cancer, she became a Survivor of a different sort: She was chosen from over 6100 applicants to participate in the very first season of CBS's history-making show, "Survivor". She has put her celebrity status to good use, appearing at charity events and speaking about cancer survival around the country. She is a national example of one who has re-channeled life's challenge into encouragement and meaning for others. banjosonja@comcast.net*

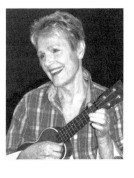

I f you will imagine for a moment the following scene—or, if you were watching the 2000 premiere of the very first episode of the controversial new reality television show, *Survivor,* you may recall the image:

It is night in a dark, humid jungle on a deserted island 5 degrees above the equator someplace in the South China Sea. Eight of us have hiked 1-1/2 hours over tortuous trails, in the rain, having been stopped twice by encounters with six-foot poisonous snakes across our path. We are now sitting around a cauldron of fire, the yellowish, smoky light from surrounding tiki torches dancing off our sweaty faces.

You can feel the tension: After three days living as castaways, the Tagi tribe is about to vote off one of its members, and—though you have no real awareness of it at the time—later, over 51 million Americans will view this scene as it is played again and again on national television: Whoever gets the most votes from their tribe members will carry with them forever the dubious distinction of being "the first Survivor voted off the island".

Macabre interest is further heightened by the fact that in the original Swedish version of *Survivor* the first one voted off went home and took his life.

WHO on earth, and in their right minds, would subject themselves to the possibility of such public humiliation? And WHY? Why would ANY one, let alone a nice, 60-something-year old girl like me, take on such an adventure in the first place?

Here's how I summed it up for CBS in my audition tape:

"I would welcome the opportunity to be your Ultimate Survivor. I wouldn't be doing it just for me—I already am a survivor—but I'd be doing it for the other Seniors out there, looking to redefine what it means to age, and for the millions of women fighting and surviving breast cancer. I sure wouldn't want to let 'em down. See you on Pulau Tiga!"

In just over a month after submitting that tape, I was amazed to learn I had made the first cut and was now one of 800 people around the country they wanted to interview further. They were looking for people who were "strong-willed, outgoing, adventurous, physically and mentally adept, adaptable to new environments, interesting lifestyles, backgrounds and personalities!"

"What an interesting group of people to share an adventure with!" I thought. "And think of the stories I could tell my grandchildren". (Actually, I didn't have any, but, if I did... think of it!) "And I could lose weight!" A psychologist friend of mine said of my reasons for wanting to do *Survivor,* "Sonja, you are the perfect mix of optimism and denial".

But now, learning that I was being seriously considered, I began to have second thoughts. Could I, albeit a former athlete, hold up physically? What about the very real health risks of insect-borne disease and slow-to-heal infections in the tropics, of particular concern to someone at risk for lymphodema since breast cancer surgery? Reports of poisonous snakes and four-foot monitor lizards worried me less than wondering if I could get my arthritic body up off the sand in the middle of the night to answer nature's call. Would prize money of one million dollars make it become a mean-spirited experience?

Friends and family were less than encouraging, fearing for my physical safety and possible exploitation by the television network.

Try as I may, however, I could not shake the seductive lure of the chance to live out a childhood fantasy I'd had since seeing Swiss Family Robinson in the movies 50-some years earlier. My ambivalence escalated: Wisdom dictated I drop out, but the feelings in my heart kept prevailing.

Something else seemed to be propelling me, something beyond its being about my love of adventure, my testing my live-off-the-land farm girl know-how, and my Robinson Crusoe spirit, something more than my getting an all-expense paid vacation on a tropical island half way around the world where I wouldn't have to take a camera or send postcards to share it with my friends! No, applying for this had everything to do with my OWN survival.

Not quite two years before, I had been diagnosed with invasive breast cancer with a 5-cm. tumor (approximately 2 inches). An important footnote here: My internist had previously told me that since I had NO history of cancer in my family, I could wait and get a mammogram every TWO years, if I chose, instead of annually. So, being a busy and healthy person, I chose to wait. Two years to the month from my previous mammogram, I discovered that when I lifted my left breast a lateral crease appeared across it. I knew this wasn't normal, but I just figured it would go away... just as would the phenomenon of my left breast beginning to outgrow my bra on that side. A week or two later, it hadn't gone away, and I went to my doctor. Things moved very fast from there, and soon I received that shocking, gut-wrenching, benumbing diagnosis that happens only to other people.

The weeks and months that followed might be characterized, in the words of Charles Dickens, as "The best of times and the worst of times". The "Best" part might include getting a glimpse of, at a really gut level, just how precious—how finite—life is, thereby gracing me with the opportunity to live it with fuller awareness. A breast cancer survivor in Ogden, Utah, where I was speaking came up afterwards and handed me a piece of paper on which was written:

*Every morning God quietly and routinely pours another 24 hours of existence into our small, cupped hands.*

*We, so dazed and benumbed by its everlasting regularity, are careless—letting slip some the precious moments He has given.*

*Most often we take the day for granted without realizing it was never promised, never put into a contract, never guaranteed.*

*–P.C. Brownlow*

Cancer can be a wake-up call.

Another "Best" during those times was the unbelievable outpouring of love and support by friends, church members, healthcare professionals, and even complete strangers --those angels who, with their financial contributions and/or volunteerism, provide more services, more comfort, more hope, than they probably ever will know.

The "Worst" of times, of course, included the endless doctors visits and treatments, surgery, and the side effects of chemotherapy and radiation.

However, in true survivor fashion, in partnership with the medical community, for the next six months, I focused my mind and energies on beating cancer.

My treatment included an aggressive regime of neoadjuvant chemotherapy followed by lumpectomy, lymph-node dissection, and 37 treatments of radiation. Some of my personal coping mechanisms included (1) learning everything I could through reading and talking with others (just my own way of trying to gain some semblance of control out of an otherwise out-of-control situation); (2) joining a support group and availing myself of the services of other cancer support organizations; (3) thinking positively about the outcome, and reinforcing this by listening to tapes and attending a symposium where speakers inspired us to not only to survive, but to THRIVE; (4) remaining socially and physically active; (5) making nutritionally conscious food choices, as well as taking appropriate vitamins and supplements and (6) last, but certainly not least, keeping a sense of humor, black though it became at times! (I'm reminded of Oscar Wilde who, on his deathbed in Paris, gazed at the ceiling and sighed: "That wallpaper is awful. One of us has to go.")

What else could I do but laugh at this one: Right after I was diagnosed, which was in December, I heard about a new book out called *"A Year to Live"* by Stephen Levine—the idea being that if we can wrap our minds around the fact that life is limited, we can live it more meaningfully and prepare better for our ultimate departure. Thinking it might give me some direction, I went to the bookstore, which didn't have it in yet but would order it. A week or so later, a young clerk called me and said, "The book you ordered, *'A Year to Live?'* It won't be in till April!"

But sometimes the fallout from serious illness can have far-reaching consequences on families that are not so laughable—in my case it was having to end a long and loving relationship when trust was shattered upon learning my partner was having an "inappropriate relationship" with someone at the workplace during the time I was most debilitated by cancer treatment. This was ultimately more devastating and life changing than the cancer itself. Try as we may, time proved that without trust, love is not enough. During the last four months of treatment, I managed to put on a brave front, but the heartache of the secret I harbored took its toll: By the time we separated, a year after my diagnosis, I was physically, emotionally and spiritually exhausted. So at age 62, having to give up a lovely home and find another place to live, I moved to a retirement community to live out my so-called "golden years".

Even though I threw myself into all kinds of activities and tried to present a positive image, it seemed no amount of diversion, or therapy, or support from friends could help me make sense of what had happened... I felt SO betrayed! I kept searching for the insight or understanding that would provide that magic bullet to kill the pain that was eating at my heart, fueled by grief and anger. Everything I read or heard told me that the path to true healing would be through forgiveness. But how do you do that? Forgiving felt like I was saying what happened was O.K., and I couldn't feel that way.

Yet eventually I realized that if I kept recreating the pain of the past in the present, I would be creating a future just like the past! In a desperate attempt to find peace, I finally was forced to search beyond the tools of intellectual and psychological insight, and to open myself to new spiritual exploration and practice.

"As a man thinketh, so he shall be," it says in the Bible. So, putting it simply, I began to practice new ways of "thinketh". I finally found a definition of forgiveness that I could accept and embrace: In her book, *A Return to Love*, Marianne Williamson says, "Forgiveness is 'selective remembering'—a conscious decision, a choice, to see things as they are NOW and let the rest go". From Dr. Fred Luskin's book, *Forgiving for Good: Holding a Grudge is Hazardous to your Health*, I learned that forgiving is not about condoning, or accepting, or forgetting, or reconciliation. "Forgiveness is the feeling of peace that emerges as you take your hurt less personally... and take responsibility for how you feel. Forgiveness is for you and no one else. Forgiveness means that even though you are wounded you choose to hurt and suffer less."

At first I thought that approach smacked of Pollyanna or self-delusion, but I was tired of hurting—of giving so much power to something that happened in the past! So when painful memories got triggered, instead of chewing on them to justify rather than heal the wound, I would consciously try to replace or block them with other, more positive thoughts or by repeating what sometimes could seem like a meaningless mantra... "I forgive you, and surrender you to a higher power. I forgive you and surrender you." The painful moments became further and further apart.

As I tried to focus on my blessings rather than my misfortunes, and reach out to others in my own need to heal, an amazing series of serendipitous opportunities began to occur, one of which was an invitation to the Women's Outdoor Adventure Training Camp in Southern California which opened its doors for one weekend to 18 breast cancer survivors from around the country. For three days, we were trained in rock climbing, mountain biking, kayaking and orienteering. Though considerably older than the other 17 participants, I launched myself fearlessly (some might say "recklessly") into the Outward Bound type of experience. On the last day, I was told by the young staff that I had so frightened them hurtling down hills on a mountain bike, or dangling from ropes on a rock face, that they were considering removing me for my own safety!

I may have terrified the staff, but the other young participants struggling with their own recovery and fears about longevity seemed to take heart seeing someone older who, despite cancer, could live a full and vital life. On the plane flying home—whether because of the headiness of the altitude or the glass of Chardonnay—I had two revelations, both of which would color the course of my life.

One was that our survivorship, whether from cancer or anything else, is not just about our own healing but it's also about the hope we can give others by our example and modeling. The second discovery was that I could still do physically demanding things.

It was with that realization that, when I returned home and read in the newspaper that CBS was looking for 16 Americans to cast away on a deserted island and see who could survive, I decided to go for it! Oh, I knew I'd never be chosen, but I also knew that if I didn't apply I would regret it. Thanks to the wake-up call of cancer, regrets were what I didn't want to have when I reached the end of life, so, just to "get it out of my system," I sent in a tape.

Well, the rest, as they say, is history. I was told my tape caught the eye of the President of CBS, so—along with 48 other finalists—I was flown to Los Angeles; after eight days of psychological testing, medical review and interviews on- and off-camera, I was selected. Five weeks later, along with the clothes on my back and ukulele as my one "luxury item", I was flown half way round the world, taken out on a fishing boat and dumped somewhere in the middle of South China Sea to swim for 2-1/2 hours pushing a raft with my tribe to a deserted island beach to try to survive for 39 days. Was I scared? Heavens no. Anyone who's been through chemotherapy and radiation can do anything for 39 days!

After three days of hard work, intense heat, and eating nothing but raw coconut and a little seaweed, I fell in the first Immunity Challenge and went on to become that First Person Ever Voted off *Survivor*—a dubious distinction at best, but ripe for a Trivial Pursuit question I am told.

What a journey—from survivor to *Survivor—and,* from survivor to thriver! Talk about lemons turning into lemonade. Along the way I learned one of the most important lessons of my life, that of forgiveness, but, most remarkably, this adventure has provided a platform from which I can give back to others the hope and support that was given to me.

Would I change any of it? Unequivocally, no.

In conclusion, I would like to contrast my two survival experiences ... that of a castaway and that of a cancer patient:

*Rats running over you at night?* Hey, I'd take this any day over a
diagnosis of a potential killer running through me!

*Privacy invaded by those ever-present TV cameras?* What about
those frequent medical exams where strange hands pat and probe areas
usually reserved for... well, those who at least take us to dinner first?

*Poisonous snakes on the island?* I remember a liquid poison snaking
from an I.V. into my arm—potentially lifesaving, but oh those side effects...

*Dirty hair and no shampoo?* Try no hair.

*Not enough to eat?* How about not being able to eat—or gagging when you try?

*Hot weather and dry skin?* If you're woman on chemo, try hot flashes and dry everything else!

*Painful sunburn?* Very much like radiation burn!

*Being the first one voted off the island?* Compared to REAL survival, it was a piece of cake! We know who the real heroes are and it has nothing to do with getting on television.

As for my own journey with cancer, I would close with the words of Sarah Mores Campbell: "We receive fragments of holiness, glimpses of eternity, brief moments of insight. Let us gather them up the precious gifts that they are, and, renewed by their grace, move boldly into the unknown."

# 9.
# Be The Change

## BY ANDREA COOMANS

*Andrea Coomans lives with her fabulous husband, Peter, and their three gorgeous sons in Salt Lake City, Utah. Andrea has a bachelors degree and a masters degree in prosthetics and currently works as an account manager for Amoena US corporation. Andrea.Coomans@amoena.com*

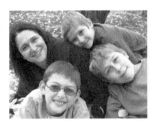

I was beginning a three week vacation in Germany when I found a lump in my left breast. After three weeks of wondering about the lump, my vacation was finally over and I could schedule an appointment with a doctor and find out what this lump was. When I was examined, the doctor said very matter of fact "Any history of breast cancer in your family?" I felt ill and couldn't fathom why he would ask me such a question. After what seemed like hundreds of appointments with several doctors, breast specialists and lastly a surgeon, I sat looking at my doctor waiting to hear the words "Everything looks fine". His mouth was moving but surely I wasn't hearing him correctly, "You need to have a mastectomy." What? Is he talking to me? Did someone walk in the room behind me? Surely he can't be talking to me, I am only 23. Yes, he is talking to me.

It was almost a three hour drive to my parent's home, but I needed to tell them that I was scheduled to have a mastectomy in two weeks. As I was driving, a black crow flew into my car and black feathers flew everywhere. I don't remember anything about the rest of the drive. I was a 23 year old career woman with no plans to marry or have children, not anytime in my future and now I was going to have mastectomy. That wasn't in my plans either.

After the initial shock, I carried on as if nothing was happening. I was very matter of fact with my surgeries, all six of them. At age 24, only seven months later, I needed my other breast removed. I still remained very calm and accepting.

I prayed, meditated, and focused on healing.

What helped me through my surgeries and experiences were many different things. I wrote a journal expressing my thoughts and feelings. I could reflect on this experience and it helped me to realize the many blessings in my life. I painted my nails bright red, fingers and toes; this helped me to feel happy and more feminine and was very psychological healing for me. I bought myself a gift before each surgery - something I might not usually buy for myself, something that felt special. I would go out to dinner the night before my surgery as a celebration of me and my life.

My life was becoming different. I began seeing things as I never remembered seeing them before—seeing things from a child's eyes and a child's wonder and joy in all things.

Part way through the processes of my second mastectomy and reconstruction surgeries I met a truly amazing man who captured my heart. He proposed a few months later and we were married a few short months after that. We moved to the United States thirteen months after our wedding which was two and half years after my initial diagnosis.

Not long after living in the United States, my silicone implants were causing extreme pain in my chest. I consulted with a plastic surgeon and was advised to remove my implants and have a tram flap reconstruction. My husband pleaded with me not to do this, but given this was my body and my decision I decided to have what I thought would be my last surgery. The surgery was fourteen hours. Too many complications occurred, even though I was a healthy 28 years old at the time. It was a nightmare experience for me. My reconstruction did not work on one side. I felt all the sadness that I should have felt at my first mastectomy. All my emotions came at me all at once.

When I came home from the hospital, my husband was emptying my drains and helping to shower me. I said "Look at me, I feel like the bride of Frankenstein" to which he replied "And I am thrilled to be Frankenstein." We laughed until we were crying.

Miraculously four months after my tram flap, I found out I was pregnant. After being told we would never have children this was an incredible blessing in our lives. Our beautiful son was born eight months later. Today, I reflect on my life. My first surgery was 19 years ago. I have been married to the most incredible man for 17 years. We miraculously have three very handsome sons who will all be taller than me in about a minute. I am very, very grateful for my diagnosis. Yes, I was 23. Yes, I had a fabulous career. But my diagnosis saved my life and taught me how to live, really and truly live. To see the joy in each day. To love being a woman. To love being a wife and a mother. To love my body as the gift it truly is.

My life changed, my body changed, my thinking changed, my life's work changed. I still want to help as many woman as I can on their journey. I feel if I could help at least one lady through her journey then mine would have been worth it.

Six years ago I started to work as an account manager for Amoena, an international company that produces and sells post surgical and breast form products for women. I travel to many states making a difference for hundreds of woman ever year. I love visiting with each of them, helping them with their post surgical garments, prostheses and, more importantly, with their well being. I share Amoena's philosophy to help make life beautiful again for all woman on this journey. When you look around, we are all different heights, different weight, different hair color, different eye color, different skin color. We all sound different and have different accents, yet we are all incredibly beautiful and are the only one of us created. One of my favorite quotes is by Mahatma Gandhi that says "Be the Change that you want to see in the world" and hopefully I am.

# 10.
# Sister Suzie Sitting on a Thistle Patch

## BY SUSAN D'AGOSTINO

*Currently Susan D'Agostino resides in White Rock, BC Canada. She is an accredited Practitioner in The Journey and a Conscious Coach. She has completed her book "Hello Susan, It's Me, Cancer!" It is available through www.healingeverybody.com.*

"Say Sister Suzie sitting on a thistle patch." He sat on a chair as his four year old daughter stood next to him. Susan's blue eyes peered into the fierce intensity of the green eyes of her father, his stern glare scaring her. She repeated the tongue twister the best she could in spite of the lisp he was so earnestly trying to correct. "I'll be dammed if one of my kids is going to go around speaking like an idiot," was his angry reasoning for this ruthless agony he was putting her through.

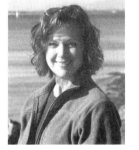

Susan knew she couldn't say her S's properly but she was desperately trying to. She didn't want to sound like an idiot, even though she wasn't quite sure what that was. She only wanted to please him and apparently she couldn't do that because she couldn't speak right. He would then repeat the phrase mimicking her and her lisp. She felt self conscious, humiliated and embarrassed. She felt small and defenseless as she tried in vain to speak right and make him happy.

So there she was condemned and humiliated at the age of four for not speaking properly. Throughout her childhood, Susan was a well behaved child and was never able to speak up for herself,

until... forty years later,

when her voice was seemingly pulled out of her during an altercation with her husband. The primal sound erupted out of her like the war cry of some unidentifiable animal. Was it a scream or a growl? Who or what was making this guttural primal sound?

As the realization set in that is was coming from HER, at first it was unfathomable, then startling. The shame that washed over and through her was too large to control. It was too great to calm. It burst forth with such intensity nothing could stand in its way; nothing could hold it back. It seemed to have a power all its own. With all this force coming so swiftly, all she could do was run for the bathroom where she could hide and cry, to shriek the anguish of four decades of pent-up torture, sadness, shame, humiliation and rage of not being heard, not being understood, and not being fully accepted.

Susan reached the point that was beyond her capacity to cope. After the tears, came the numb feeling, the feeling of nothing, floating, lightness, calm... nothing mattered... it was like being in a parallel universe.

Why wouldn't her husband listen to her? Why could he not hear her? Why did she have no voice around him?

A year earlier, Susan had been told she had breast cancer. Her husband had just begun to renovate their home when she was diagnosed. Not only was her body, mind, spirit and emotions in a state of upheaval and reconstruction, but her surroundings mirrored this as well. Nothing was in place in her life. Nothing seemed in her control anymore, her health, her marriage, her sanity, her home were all in a state of chaos. The disarray in her life, her body and her home were too big and overwhelming for Susan to deal with.

At the forefront of all of Susan's looming problems was the question of dying. When the thought of doing chemotherapy crossed her mind, this fear sucked the energy out of her body and threatened to drive her already stressed out mind to the brink of insanity. If she did chemotherapy, she was afraid it would kill her. Was she just being difficult once again, by not going along with what everybody else thought and believed? How was she going to find the people she so desperately needed to help her? It seemed that if she chose natural and alternative healing methods then she was on her own, spit out of the system like a bad tasting vegetable out of a baby's mouth.

What was she going to do? Faced with the feelings of fear, deep despair, and sadness was also an overwhelming burden of not being able to make decisions that felt best for her.

Susan asked herself, whose decision is this? She also asked herself, which was worse, taking her life in her own hands or putting her life in someone else's? How could she trust anyone when she believed the chemotherapy could possibly kill her? She repeatedly asked herself if there were other ways to heal.

The mind numbing indecision haunted her for days, until finally she decided to find the people she needed and do alternative and natural healing of this they call breast cancer. She had surgery to remove the lump one week after she had been diagnosed—there had been no time to think, let alone to consider if the surgery was in her best interest. Thank goodness she had two months to heal from the surgery before she was scheduled for eight rounds of chemotherapy followed by radiation and hormone therapy for five years.

Susan met a woman who had done alternative treatments and was an eight year living example of someone who actually healed by using alternative methods to chemotherapy. This woman shared new ideas with Susan what she might consider doing and who to ask for help. The woman also recommended Susan to take responsibility for her healing choices and to choose healing partners that felt right for her.

At first Susan felt confident that she was on her way forward until the first three naturopaths told her "they could not help her." But Susan was persistent to find someone who could serve her healing needs.

It was the fourth naturopath who finally said he had experience with cancer and helping others heal from it. She began taking Vitamin C intravenously advised by the naturopath and took the specific herbs prescribed by a herbalist. She modified her diet to include freshly squeezed vegetable juices and began to cook and eat lots of green vegetables including kale, spinach and chard. Along with her homemade vegetable soup and salads, she began taking iodine and minerals, adding them to her diet. It became important to Susan to restrict sugar as well as yeast, wheat and other grains. She also saw a specialized Kinesiologist, a medical intuitive, two different counselors and a doctor from an integrated clinic.

As time went on, Susan almost believed she could fully heal.

Little did she know this was the beginning of her healing process, she learned she also needed spiritual, emotional, and mental guidance.

Susan found comfort by taking long walks in the forest which was close by her home and some days she walked along the beach. She was mesmerized by the beauty of the forest, the magnificent trees seemed to calm her fears and doubts about whether she was healed or not. Soon, she began to gain insights about her own life; it was as if this knowledge was there to be understood by anyone accepting of it. She asked and prayed to her angels daily that she would release her nay saying thoughts and unhealthy feelings from her mind and body. Some days all she could muster up was, *"Help me, help me, help me."*

The beautiful, insightful walks in the forest always brought her to calm and peace and always a resolution for the time being. She listened to positive CD's and constantly worked on keeping good thoughts flowing which was challenging at times when she walked into the house and looked around at her home and the ugliness all around her. It was like trying to put her mind and imagination in a completely different place than she was experiencing and living in. How could she imagine feeling happy and healed when her life was so miserable? She didn't even know how to speak to her husband without making him angry and her own anger was always simmering just below the surface.

One day, they were arguing about how the house looked. Her point was that it was down right embarrassing to always be living in a mess and she threw in some points about how it was taking much too long to complete, not to mention he constantly began tearing apart another room before the previous one was complete. His response was that it was her fault how the house looked. The audacity of his statement sent her through a state of uncontrollable rage she had never felt before in her life!

Susan could feel her breath coming in great heaving gasps for air. A huge wave of energy began to work its way up her legs through the rest of her body. She began to shake violently in the torment of this incredible power. To her astonishment, she witnessed her own two hands reach out and grab him by the sweatshirt he was wearing and half pulled half dragged him up eleven plywood steps screaming at him the whole time at the outrageous comment and how in the world could it be her fault the house was in such shambles? At the top of the steps, she finally came to her senses and let him go. Stunned at what had just transpired, she ran crying to the bathroom where she sobbed for the better part of an hour. What was happening to her? How did she just drag her husband up all those steps? She could not comprehend her bizarre behavior, never before had she ever felt so unglued and so out of control, but at the same time she had never felt so free, in that moment. It was scary to feel like she had lost her mind, but on the other hand there was no turning back now, there was no escaping this radical energy that erupted out of her being at any given time.

She could feel the rage coming through her body, it was always triggered by someone aggravating her or pushing her a little too far. It was always followed by an immediate feeling of freedom, of nothing being held back, of complete release. Then the numbness, the feeling that nothing mattered, of complete surrender, not caring about anything, sometimes she sat and stared at the walls for hours, frozen in time, her arms too heavy to lift to wipe the tears streaming down her face or the snot dripping from her nose, unable to hold on to any thought in this place of nothingness. It felt like she was being pulled into blackness, the big black hole of depression she had fought so hard to stay out of throughout her lifetime.

After some hours passed, she felt herself take a breath and she came back into her body. She spent days in this state of complete and utter surrendering bliss.

Soon it became evident that the releasing of her lifelong confined emotions were making a difference in her life. She realized this one morning when she woke feeling good which had not been a consistent feeling in her life. She allowed this feeling to expand and for the first time in her life Susan embraced the feeling of being happy. Nothing had changed in her outer world, the mess and plywood were still everywhere, only now there was peace in her being. Susan had found her voice and it was saving her life. It began when she took her focus off of how badly the house looked and felt to her and she focused on how she wanted to feel. A sense of purpose was coming alive in her; Susan wanted to something she could immerse herself into and use her own experience as a living example of how the body can heal. She wanted to help others with their healing experiences.

And finally, the understanding came that she wasn't a victim. She had choices. Susan realized that her husband actually helped her to bring forth the suppressed anger that had been eating away so that she could finally release it and set it free. After all, this is what she had prayed for almost every day when she walked through the forest. Susan began to feel compassion and deep gratitude for her husband playing the part in her healing experience. She accepted him for who he was and began welcoming a softening in her heart toward him. The softening and understanding also brought forth a new sense of freedom. She no longer needed to be in control. She could accept things as they were with no expectations. Susan finally felt love, gratitude, peace and happiness.

As Susan began to feel more and more healed and whole, she wondered what work she would call her own, then one day she heard Skip Lackey conduct a tele-seminar, sharing the story how Brandon Bays personally experienced a miraculous healing. Susan instantly knew this was her calling. Soon she immersed herself into this emotional healing work called THE JOURNEY and her unhealed childhood memories began to come forth, one after another.

*The Susan I was then is not the same person I am today. I am more joy filled. I live in the present because I have healed many layers of my painful past. Thriving and being in love with life has replaced what was bubbling under my skin. I continue to meditate and spend time alone. I allow my emotions to flow through as they do and to stay focused on what I DO want in my life. I practice feeling the way I want to feel and I practice keeping quiet when I don't want to feel an emotion and letting it pass without attaching to it. I also use all the tools and skills I have learned to keep me on track in my life. Once a week I trade healing sessions with another Journey Practitioner. I want to keep myself as clear as possible so I can keep living in each moment just as I AM.*

# 11.
# Sherry Lebed Davis, Thriving After Breast Cancer

## BY BEVERLY VOTE

*Sherry Lebed Davis is a recognized authority on the use of movement and therapeutic exercise for healing and quality of life issues after breast cancer, all cancers, Lymphedema, and all chronic illness. She is the co-founder with Dr. Marc Lebed and Dr. Joel Lebed of Healthy-Steps moving you to better health with THE LEBED METHOD, a worldwide organization providing unique wellness programs for special populations. Her work has been recognized in People Magazine, Health Magazine, Oxygen, Spa Magazine, Coping, CURE, NY Times, Seattle Times, and LA Times. She has appeared on the Today Show, Life Time Live, Nightly News, BBC and many more. She presents across the United States and internationally. Sherry authored "Thriving after Breast Cancer, Essential Healing Exercises for Body and Mind" and has produced two DVDs and a musical CD. www.lebedmethod.com / info@lebedmethod.com*

*What better way to thrive than to have fun doing it!*
*–Sherry Lebed Davis*

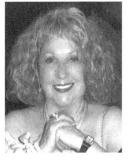

Dance movement has been used as therapy throughout the world for centuries. Dance helps us to release and express our deeper emotions, increases our sense of well-being, gives us a break from our troubles, helps shake off our lingering fears, and creates a sense that we belong. Dance continues to be used for therapy, celebration and in sacred tribal rituals around the world.

It is intriguing to see how dance in the life of Sherry Lebed Davis brought her to a place that makes a huge impact for those facing breast cancer. It began with Sherry's heartfelt desire to help her mother when her mother was diagnosed with breast cancer. But the story doesn't end there, nor did it begin there: When Sherry was diagnosed with breast cancer, she experienced the benefit of the very program she designed for her mother, and once again, from someplace deep in her heart, Sherry knew she wanted to help people all around the world with the program that turned out to be the therapy her mom needed. The love of movement and music was first cultivated by Sherry's mom and today Sherry cultivates the love of movement in dance in others.

Sherry Lebed Davis' journey with breast cancer began with a family history of the disease. Her grandmother and two aunts had breast cancer and, in 1980, her mother was diagnosed. Although her mother was treated successfully, her recovery had many challenges, both physically and emotionally. Sherry's desire to bring a smile back to her mother's face spawned a program and a business that now aids recovery for thousands of participants worldwide.

Both of Sherry's parents were professional ballroom dancers and their home was filled with music and dance. In Sherry's adult life, she too became a professional dancer. Her two brothers chose to be surgeons. Because Sherry and her brothers grew up in an environment that believed music and dance were beneficial components for healing body and mind, it felt natural for the Lebed siblings to design something special for their mother based on movement, music and medical methodology.

Their goal was to improve their mother's physical range of motion, increase flexibility, improve balance, strength, and endurance, and bolster her emotional well-being and self-image and have fun doing it. Their mother was soon smiling again and her physical recovery improved after employing the program that was designed specifically for her by her children.

In 1996, Sherry was diagnosed and treated for breast cancer. Sherry used the same program she helped develop for her mother. While in the midst of her own treatment and recovery, she was determined to help as many survivors as possible by teaching the program, 'Lebed Method', at local hospitals in the Seattle area. Along the way, Sherry wrote a book Thriving after Breast Cancer: Essential Healing Exercises for Body and Mind, and filmed two DVD's for home use.

The head of a breast cancer center at a major hospital in Philadelphia saw the need for the Lebed family program and soon adopted it into therapy for their patients. From that program evolved the first of four medical studies on the Lebed Method, quantifying its effect on recovery and quality of life. Today, the program is currently in over 800 hospitals, community centers, and fitness centers and in 14 countries. "It is fulfilling and gratifying to see the wonderful benefits of our recovery program, known as Healthy-Steps: moving you to better health with the Lebed Method, helping so many across the country and internationally," said Sherry.

Healthy-Steps is a fun program where the movement and music are the mediums through which one experiences therapeutic exercise. Playful props, such as boas, bubbles, and scarves are used to make the exercises enjoyable and fun. No certain level of physical or dance ability is required. Chairs are provided for anyone who may wish to participate seated. Healthy-Steps is not an aerobic type program, so the people who attend the classes vary in ages and physical conditions. It is strongly advised that if a participant experiences any pain during an exercise, they are encouraged to stop or ratchet their efforts back. Healthy Steps teaches "No pain means more gain." The exercises are designed to be gentle resistance so everyone can do them according to their ability. There is no competition. As with any exercise program, all participants are encouraged to consult their physician before beginning.

With Healthy-Steps:
- There is no need to know how to dance to receive benefit from this program.
- Participants do not feel self-conscious and they can start at any stage of their healing journey knowing that this program does not harm them.
- Physical strength and lung capacity are benefited.

- Everyone's spirits are lifted. Originally developed to aid recovery for breast cancer survivors, Healthy-Steps classes are now benefiting participants who are dealing with a broad range of conditions from other cancers, lymphedema, multiple sclerosis, arthritis, Parkinson's, chronic fatigue syndrome, and fibromyalgia to name a few.

The original program has been adapted for aquatic exercises, maternity programs, senior health and wellness and children undergoing treatment or dealing with chronic illness. "My brothers and I developed our program to empower our mother with the knowledge that her recovery could be in her own hands. She did not need to feel as though she was powerless and at the hands of a whimsy-less fate. Once she started incorporating what she loved to do which was to move to music, she regained her emotional equilibrium and that helped power her physical recovery as did mine," said Sherry.

"We as breast cancer survivors have psychological and physical scars that need to be addressed. After a diagnosis of breast cancer or any chronic condition, we need to feel we can and are doing something for ourselves—something we enjoy, that is pleasurable and that gives us results we can feel. I know this program meets all those needs and that is why I continue even with all my traveling to teach several Healthy-Steps classes a week myself so I can continue to know surviving is important but thriving is elegant. Smiles and laughter all around in our classes show me our program succeeds in our goals and in our attendees' goals."

"Empowerment to take charge of one's recovery need not be a lonely quest. By sharing and encouraging each other, we build a stronger foundation for continued recovery.

And what better way to thrive than to have fun doing it!" said Sherry.

# 12.

# Cancer Gave Me Courage to Thrive

## BY PAULA HOLLAND DE LONG, CPCC, ACC

*Cancer thriver, certified life coach, author, and speaker Paula Holland De Long CPCC, ACC, is an authority on how the lessons of survivorship can bring joy, passion and purpose to anyone's life. Her first book, the 'What's Next For My Life? Companion Journal for Cancer Patients' has just been published and second book is coming soon. Her workshops and classes are offered at cancer treatment centers and support organizations. Her teleconference groups attract participants from around the country. Paula is President of What's Next For My Life, Inc. Phone: 954-565-6894 www.WhatsNextForMyLife.com*

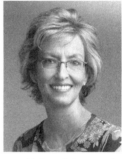

**B**efore cancer, I thought I was successful but I was dying inside. Coming face to face with my own mortality changed everything. That was in 1996. Cancer took away my marriage and led me to my soul mate. Cancer forced me to admit that I hated my career and inspired me leave it and pursue my passion. Cancer gave me the strength to truly believe that I could do anything and gave me the gift of allowing people to help me to do it.

I was diagnosed with breast cancer when I was 37. Terrified and not knowing what was next for my life, my shock and disbelief had barely sunk in before I was living it. I was living a normal life and four weeks later I was in a hospital minus my left breast and wondering what was next for my life.

Overwhelmed by pain and fear, wondering how this could be happening to me, I put one foot in front of the other during chemotherapy. I kept my "I'm fine" face on and my wig straight in 90 degree heat and 90% humidity. I tried to be superwoman even when I could barely get out of bed. I waited for that magic time when the cancer stuff would end and I could go back to "normal."

My surgeries and treatment finally ended. Everyone was so thrilled that I was "done" with cancer. But I wasn't. Even though the GI Jane hair looked good, I was exhausted and weighed 95 pounds with scars all over. I was afraid of the cancer coming back. I felt so different from before I thought I was sure I had a brain tumor. I didn't.

Feeling raw, afraid, and uncertain, my femininity, confidence, and belief in who I was had been stripped away by cancer. The voices in my head were telling me "No one will ever want you again because of the scars. You're too sick to do anything. Your life is over," and, "You're going to be sad forever."

Some serious soul searching began. I thought about things which brought me down, zapped my energy, and made me feel bad about myself. I had so many negatives in my life.

I knew beyond a shadow of a doubt that my old life had made me sick. I knew in my heart I had to change and try some new ways of living and being.

I started focusing on things that made me feel good, made me feel alive, things I was drawn to. Being outside every day, enjoying time with the people I loved, and singing out loud to my favorite songs brought me back to life. I began letting go of things that I HAD to do or SHOULD be done. I gave myself permission to listen to my heart.

Instead of going back to my high stress executive position I decided to take a lower paying, mid-level job. I started gardening and walking the dog. Soon my husband was asking me "Who are you and what have you done with Paula?" (He didn't mean that in a positive way). I was feeling better, but I still kept wondering "what's next for my life?" and feeling "there's got to be more." Connecting with other survivors was the next step in my journey to thriving. When I was trained as a volunteer to visit newly diagnosed women, suddenly I wasn't alone with my cancer anymore. Women who understood the big and little things that I was struggling with told me I could get a prosthesis to fill up the empty hole in my bra. They taught me my frustration with my old life was okay. They gave me the courage to say "no" to negativity and "yes" to choosing a happy, joyful future on my own terms. They taught me to give back. Their strength, compassion and honesty opened my heart in a way I had never felt before.

I began visiting several newly diagnosed women every week. I could see their faces light up when their eyes inevitably went to my chest and my smile. When we met they were fearful, lonely and afraid. We were smiling and hugging each other when I left. They gained hope from my recovery. My confidence grew as I helped them. My thriving quotient went up. But I still didn't know who I was.

My husband and I had grown apart, and my job, although less stressful, left me empty and unfulfilled. I took the next biggest leap of faith of my life. Over a four month period my husband and I parted (amicably); I gave notice to my job; bought my own house; and started my own company. Everyone thought I was crazy or having a mid life crisis, and maybe I was. I did know in my heart and my soul that I was doing what I was meant to do and I was powerless to deny it.

So there I was. No husband, no clients, and a looming mortgage payment. The voices in my head were screaming things like "You're too old to start over. You only have one breast; no one will want ever you again," and "you're going to fail and be living in your car." I was shocked when my previous employer became my first client because I had gathered up my courage and asked. The "before cancer Paula" would have been afraid to try. I had followed my heart and successfully created my own company! I was exhilarated and my confidence grew.

Soon I had a wonderful new man in my life. When I told Chuck about my breast cancer, he took my hand, put it to his heart and said "I don't care. I love all of you just the way you are." Before long, we were married. I was thriving in ways that had never been possible before my diagnosis. Before cancer I was an overworked, overstressed Type-A person who had no appreciation for anything. I was crystal clear and very vocal about what didn't work, what was wrong with my life, or other people's choices. Unknowingly, I had been living my life as a victim.

Cancer was transforming me into a woman of choice, gratefulness, and joy.

A new passion was calling my name. As I supported others struggling with the emotional and practical realities of the disease, I realized they too were truly changed emotionally and spiritually. Cancer awakened an urgent need to make the most of each day, and to give back to others. It was the "how" of doing it that challenged them. I knew in my heart that I was meant to help. I was drawn to an emerging field called life coaching, realizing coaching was a powerful tool for starting over and making changes. Learning to focus on what matters most, not what society or others think happiness should be. This idea was really resonant with me.

At my very first coach training, I knew that helping survivors understand that their emotions were normal, and teaching them how to live based on what matters most was my new professional calling. I began sharing my story and bringing workshops to cancer treatment centers and support organizations. Survivor after survivor reported huge increases in their feelings of acceptance, personal empowerment, and ability to make decisions and take action.

Once again, my faith and passion were expanded, and my happiness and gratitude soared. I was thriving and loving every minute of it. My company, What's Next For My Life, Inc. was launched. My connection with my higher power was growing. My life was more balanced between work, love, giving back and having fun than ever before.

The last few years have been the happiest of my life. I'm still working with survivors and finding new ways to support them. I believe that cancer is a wake up call, a reminder that thriving is about being our own authentic selves, and actively working to make the world a better place, one small or large step at a time.

My mantra has become, "Why wait and why worry?" My courage is based on the absolute conviction that if I can do cancer, I can do anything. My new-found way of showing up in the world is based on compassion for myself and others, with excitement and curiosity about what we can do together, rather than alone.

Dealing with cancer and all of the changes it forced on me inspired me to contribute to the world instead of standing on the sidelines. It wasn't easy. It was definitely worth it. I'm thriving now!

As I finish writing this story, I'm singing out loud to one of my favorite songs. The line that resonates in my heart says "I can be myself now finally, in fact there's nothing I can't be." I wish this for each and every one of you.

BreastCancerWellness.org

# 13.
# I am able to give back, and that makes me whole again!

## BY KATHY DIBBEN

*Kathy Dibben lives in Smithville, Missouri with her husband Bud, and a spoiled black lab named Mac. Bud and Kathy blended their families over 30 years ago. Together they have 5 children, 10 grandchildren, and a new great-grandson. She is a two time breast cancer survivor, became a certified mastectomy fitter and gives back through her appearance center, Absolute Dignity. You can contact Kathy at absolutedignity@aol.com , www.absolutedignity.com, or reach out to her on facebook.*

Being a breast cancer thriver means I am whole again. Do I have a complete body that includes breasts? No, I do not, but in my mind and in my spirit I am a whole, complete, and fulfilled woman. When I look in a mirror, I still see me.

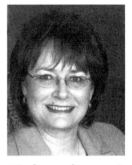

I am surrounded by a loving husband, children, grand-children, father, brother, sisters-in-law, and amazing friends. I have always had a strong family support system. I took that support for granted until my mother was diagnosed with breast cancer in 1973 and passed away with a metastasis to the bones in l983. She lived 51 years. She was a strong, petite little woman with the determination to beat this awful disease. Her attitude was always positive and she fought the battle until the very end. She empowered me to fight as well. I was diagnosed seven years after her death.

You can imagine how emotional it was for my family to hear that we had another diagnosis of breast cancer in the family. Actually, I was the third diagnosis. One week before I was told I had breast cancer, my cousin, Ann, was also diagnosed. We went through treatments together—two weeks apart. We both had the same number of chemotherapy rounds and the same number of radiation treatments. We both were advised, based on data, that we had a 25 percent chance of surviving 5 years if we underwent treatment. Ann survived two years and I am still here 20 years later.

When diagnosed, I, like so many others facing a crisis, reached for my Bible for comfort. The verse that stuck with me and that I claimed for myself during this trial, was Psalms 46:10. "Be still and know that I am God." My inner strength came from that verse telling me to be still, listen to the doctors, listen to your own body, follow their instructions, don't worry, because God was in control. Did I sometimes worry? Yes, of course I did. Mainly I worried for my family. It was harder for them at times than it was for me. I was the one sick, and they were the ones that were not sure what to do to help. When I felt discouraged or worried, I would try to think positive thoughts, go to a calming place in my mind, and always remind myself of the scripture.

The hardest thing for me to do was accept the different acts of kindness I was receiving from family and total strangers. I was trying so hard to stay in control. My life seemed to be totally in the hands of others. My experiences with breast cancer taught me to be able to receive. I had always been the one giving. I learned that allowing family and friends to help, whether it is a new hat, a new magazine, or a new step-mother chauffeuring you to treatments, is a gift that you can give to them. They feel helpless. You can continue your giving spirit by allowing others to do what they can for you.

I learned this lesson 20 years ago. I had finished chemotherapy, and 30 radiation treatments. I was to take 7 additional radiation treatments at a downtown hospital that used a different machine. I was instructed to check in at the hospital and they would direct me to the proper building for treatment.

I forgot to ask about parking. I drove a full size van at the time. There was no parking available on the streets, and the garage parking signs all said "no vans". Cars were honking at me because I was driving so slow trying to find a parking spot. I pulled into an open lot and read signs that said "private parking only, violators will be towed". I was so upset and frustrated. I just sat there and totally lost it. I had not truly let go of my emotions throughout this ordeal. The last time I had cried was seven months earlier when my hair slid off onto the pillow.

I finally pulled myself together and did find a legal parking spot. I went into the hospital and got in a line to check in. A very rude young woman yelled at me when I told her why I was there and pointed to the correct line for me. When it was my turn, I sat down at the window where a beautiful woman with true compassion and kindness began to take my information. This woman commented that I looked upset. I explained the parking situation and she just smiled and patted my hand. She was one of the largest women I have ever met. She was so large that her body covered the entire window area and blocked the view of everything behind her.

She got up to make copies of my insurance cards, and there it was... my affirmation. Behind her, was a gold plaque that read "Be still, and know that I am God" Psalms 46:10. I knew from that very second on that I truly was going to survive and later I learned to totally thrive.

When treatments were over, I had an overwhelming need to help others get through their own cancer journey. I did not belong to a support group back then, but I had many women who showed up in my path with questions or needing comfort.

Sometimes we met at a doctor appointment and began talking. Sometimes a friend of a friend of a friend would reach out to me. One time, my husband and I were in a restaurant. I noticed a young woman with small children having a really bad day. She had lost her hair, was wearing a bandana, and you could see that she was miserable. I got up to go to the restroom.

When I returned, her husband had left the table and the chair next to her was empty. Her parents and children were still at the table. I don't know what came over me, it was so unlike me, (at that time) but I just sat down in that empty chair. I asked her if she was undergoing chemo? She said yes. I asked her where her cancer was found? She said breast.

I told her I was a five year breast cancer survivor. I gave her a hug and told her it would get easier, that she was going to be okay. We both cried, and I went back to my table.

Three years later I was talking to a customer at my place of employment. She asked me if I had talked to a cancer patient a few years ago in a restaurant. I thought for a minute, and said yes. She stared at me and said "that was me! I didn't know who you were or where to find you but you gave me the strength I needed and hope."

She said her family was very supportive and they had tried to tell her she would be okay, but she said she was feeling angry and was sitting there thinking what do they know, they haven't been through this... and then you sat down.

Her words were like winning the lottery for me. I knew I was supposed to be passing out Hope!

I guess I am a slow learner or a rebellious follower. It took me 17 years from the first diagnosis of breast cancer and 5 years from the second time around to finally follow my heart and open a store that would help others through their journey. After all these years, I am now reaching women daily who need hope and encouragement. I have grown in my faith and I became a stronger person. My healing and my joy continue as I surround myself with amazing women. Some are newly diagnosed, and some had surgery more than 30 years ago.

I still know how to "be still" when I need to be. All of these women have their own story, and they need to be heard. Yes, I have had breast cancer, and I am a survivor, but even more important, I am a thriver. I have seen miracles. I am able to give back, and that makes me whole again!

# 14.

# Another Chance at Life

## BY LEONORE H. DVORKIN

*Leonore H. Dvorkin and her husband, David Dvorkin, live in Denver, Colorado. Leonore works as a tutor of Spanish and German, a proofreader and editor, a German to English translator, and a weight training instructor. Her two books are 'Another Chance at Life: A Breast Cancer Survivor's Journey' (Norilana Books, 2009 and Smashwords.com, 2010) and the novel 'Apart from You' (CreateSpace, 2010). leonore@csd.net / www.dvorkin.com*

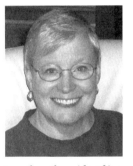

I was thrilled and honored when Beverly Vote invited me to contribute to this *Breast Cancer Thrivers* book project. What a worthy goal, I thought, and what a wonderful title—exactly in line with my thinking about what having breast cancer meant to me, how it changed my life for the better.

Among Beverly's suggested topics, I saw many that I had addressed in my own breast cancer book, *Another Chance at Life: A Breast Cancer Survivor's Journey,* which I wrote after I had breast cancer and a mastectomy in 1998. I could think of no better way to tell the readers of this current book about what my breast cancer experience meant to me—how I came out on the other side of it a better, wiser, and happier person—than to take a few excerpts from that previous book. They sum up the main events and realizations that gradually brought me to this new, very positive state: that of being a true breast cancer thriver.

In the seven selections which follow, I tell you my reasons for writing my breast cancer book; how and why my husband and I documented the changes in my body with photos; how I learned that other people cared deeply about me; how learning to accept my cancer fate gave me a more philosophical outlook on life in general; how I realized that there are many things I miss more than I miss my left breast; how my husband and I dealt with and then moved beyond the fear we both felt when I contracted cancer; and how cancer helped me lose my previous dread of growing older and gave me a deeper appreciation of life in general.

For the vast majority of us who have weathered the experience of breast cancer and breast cancer surgery, every subsequent year of good health that passes brings more relief and optimism. So I want to say, as encouragingly as I can, to any woman who is currently plagued by fear concerning her own health: Try not to worry too much! Where there is still life, there should also be hope. My heartfelt hope for you is that someday your fear and pain, like mine, will be just a memory.

For those of you who are having to deal with the myriad problems of aging as well as any necessary adjustments to cancer, I want to add the following message.

Somewhere along my own cancer journey, I realized that I had passed a significant milestone on the path of adjustment to middle age. I saw that dealing with and conquering my cancer had served as a catalyst for the acceptance of numerous other less-than-pleasant changes that were to come well after my mastectomy. With that acceptance came a wonderful new peace, accompanied by a much deeper appreciation of all the goodness and beauty in life.

About seven or eight years after my mastectomy, I became aware that the cancer experience had brought me something else, too, something that has benefited me greatly ever since. It was an intriguing and envigorating sense of courage, the courage to open myself to new experiences, to accept new professional opportunities if they should come my way. Then, as if on cue, several did!

Today, at 64, I remain very active with the work I've been doing for decades: writing, tutoring Spanish and German, translating, and teaching weight training. But in the past few years, I've added instruction in ESL (English as a Second Language) and editing for other authors. Interestingly, it was my breast cancer book that led several of my editing clients to me. The editing is bringing me tremendous satisfaction, as well as an exciting sense of discovery. I feel privileged to be gleaning some of the wide-ranging knowledge of these other writers and to be sharing in their experiences, so different from my own.

The authors who have sought me out are a diverse group. One is a young Pakistani essayist, book reviewer, and short story writer. Another man, blind from birth, writes marvelous children's books filled with adventure, optimism, and messages of the value of friendship and kindness. I'm helping a prostate cancer survivor finish a very compassionate book on intimacy after breast cancer and various gynecological cancers.

My current German to English translation project, my longest to date, is a gripping nonfiction book by a German woman who was a 19-year-old hijacking hostage in 1977. She and her fellow passengers endured five days of terror and brutality before they were rescued in Mogadishu.

All these people have overcome tremendous personal challenges, and I feel truly honored to be helping them bring their valuable messages to the world. Working with them has added new purpose and passion to my own life, and I treasure the long-distance friendships we have developed.

Here is yet another wonderful result of my breast cancer experience. In response to my book, I've received numerous e-mail letters from other breast cancer survivors in several countries: in the U.S., England, Australia, and Sweden. Reading their heartfelt messages to me, as well as some details of their own cancer experiences, has made me feel part of a very special group of women all over the world.

Thank you again, Beverly, for allowing me to be part of this book. May it bring help, hope, and encouragement to many thousands of women and their loved ones in many countries!

## From the Introduction to Another Chance at Life

I want to state at the outset that I in no way intend to say to other breast cancer survivors or patients: "This is the way you should feel. This is the way you should react. This is the path of treatment you should select." Absolutely not! Your emotions and reactions and medical choices are your own.

If my words can be of help and encouragement to other women who have gone through the experience of breast cancer or who are going through it now, then that will be a rich reward. However, this book is also for the many women who have not yet developed breast cancer but who will in the future, as well as for all the others who fear they might develop it. What I most want to tell them is that breast cancer does not have to be counted among the greatest traumas of their lives. Instead, it is entirely possible that they can go on living and doing all they did before. They can come out on the other side of the experience better than they were before, both healthier and happier.

I know this is true, because it happened to me. What follows here is the story of how.

## The Photos

The evening before my mastectomy, David and I went out and bought a Polaroid camera. We did not yet own a digital camera, and we knew that no commercial lab would develop the photos I wanted him to take: pictures of my naked body, whole for the last time. I wanted not just memories of that body, but clear and lasting evidence of the old image of myself.

In the photos, there is no sign of the disease itself. Nor is there any sign of the fear and uncertainty I felt.

The simple, grainy little pictures that resulted from that evening's photo shoot would never pass as art. We made no effort to glamorize or soften the images in any way, to make me look like anything other than the middle-aged, somewhat overweight woman I was and still am. I simply stood there unclothed, in the bathroom and then in the hallway, and let my beloved husband and the technological wonder in his hands capture my Before, the body he had known and loved for over thirty years.

That evening, neither one of us had any firm idea of what the After would look or feel like, or how either one of us would react to the changes. And so both of us wanted those pictures, evidence of how I was on that side of a great divide in my self-image and my life.

Photos of my post-surgery body would come later. Somehow, we wanted and needed to document the entire process.

There are the pictures taken the night before the surgery. There's one of the thick bandages and the drain tube and its attached bulb that I had in me and on me for three days after the surgery. There are pictures of my body freed from the bandages, unflinching pictures of my naked chest and its big red scar.

Then, two years later, came photos of my chest all healed, my body several pounds heavier but quite strong again—and my broad smile, reflecting my new joy and inner peace.

## Revelations of Affection

I was discharged from the hospital at 10:00 a.m. I bought a cappuccino in the lobby, said goodbye to the friendly nurse who waited with me while David retrieved the car, and was on my way home.

That afternoon, I received several long-distance phone calls from family members. Bouquet after bouquet of flowers arrived from far and near, from relatives and students and friends. The house soon looked like a flower shop. I was overwhelmed by the beauty, as well as by all the presents, fruit baskets, cards, phone calls, and e-mails I received. There were even some e-mails from strangers, from people whom David knew only online—other science fiction writers and readers, mainly, whom he had told about my surgery.

The cards were so numerous that I had to suspend them overlapping one another on a long string stretched across the living room hearth. They stayed there for several weeks afterward. Never in my wildest dreams could I have anticipated such an outpouring of love and concern. More than anything else, I think, that helped me to heal.

So that was the first benefit of my cancer: finding out how much other people cared about me. It was an amazing revelation.

## Fate and Philosophy

Even as I was determined to make the best of the situation, there was some residual anger that I had gotten cancer at all. I knew I had to look that anger squarely in the face and then deal with it.

A great many people besides me were surprised that I had contracted cancer. That's because anyone who knows me knows that I've worked hard, at least for most of my life, to get and stay fit and healthy. Even now, years after the end of my fulltime teaching of weight training, I eat a diet with not much fat or junk food in it. I don't smoke. I quit drinking alcohol two decades ago. I've never had hormone replacement therapy. David and I spend a great deal of money every month on vitamins, minerals, and other dietary supplements. For most of my life, I've been a model of good health habits. And it's only in recent years that I've become any more than moderately overweight.

Therefore the question remains: Why did I get cancer?

Perhaps that question will never be answered. Perhaps it cannot be answered. So, after a short while, I stopped asking it, as I found that it only irritated and depressed me. For me, it soon fell into the same category as questions about why any tragedy befalls any person. Why is one baby and not another born with crippling birth defects? Why does a given family's house get demolished by a tornado while the house next door does not? Why is a certain traveler on the highway at the same time as a certain truck driver who falls asleep at the wheel? And so on.

Sometimes there are clear answers to questions about why tragedies befall us and those we love, but usually there are not. In that case, all we can do, for the sake of our own sanity and the happiness of those around us, is accept the hand that Fate has dealt us and go on as best we can. For beyond the pain, perhaps far down the road of life, may lie some very valuable things: new knowledge of ourselves and others, new life paths to explore, and new happiness to be found.

## Other Losses in My Life

Loss. That's what we call having to give up something we value. As a woman, I can't imagine preferring to have no breasts over preferring to have two healthy ones, but I definitely wanted to be rid of my non-healthy one. For me, it was not so much a loss as it was the removal of a body part that had turned against me.

On a television program, I once heard a woman speak of feeling "mutilated" by her mastectomy. To my mind, that's a very strange term to use, as I associate it with torture. I think of mutilation as the disfiguring of a person's body done with the express purpose of causing that person pain and distress. But what could be further from the surgeon's mind? The good surgeon applies all of his or her skill toward healing, toward the removal of things that will do the body harm, toward the correction of defects caused by nature or accident.

To my mind, beneficial and necessary surgery is anything but mutilation. It may take away some of the symmetry that contributes so much to our concept of beauty. It may alter the body in ways that render it less than pleasing to look upon. But in my opinion, that's a small cost indeed for the concurrent gain in health.

What else have I lost over my lifetime that I miss more than I miss my breast? Goodness, where do I begin the list?

I miss my childhood toys, books, school papers, drawings, and paintings, all lost in the course of my family's many moves. I miss my dead grandparents, plus other people who died long before they were old. I miss my grandparents' houses in Mississippi and Louisiana, houses that are now the property of other, unrelated people. I miss various friends who either moved away or who apparently decided that our friendship was not worth maintaining. I miss our only grandchild, now a teenager, whom David and I have seen only three times in her life. (The story behind our separation does not belong here.)

I miss the ability to run without suffering pain, an ability which vanished sometime in my early teen years, when I started developing varicose veins. I miss having smooth, unscarred legs, which now, after 50 years of leg problems and five vein operations, I can barely remember. I miss modern dance classes, swimming, bicycling, and playing racquetball, all of which had to be given up for various compelling health reasons. I miss the strength and flexibility that I had before I hurt my back over twenty years ago. I miss the ease of movement and the greater physical attractiveness that came with weighing 130 pounds versus my present 195 pounds. I miss the inch of height I lost sometime during the last few years. And ever since I was first told that my bones were weakening, I've missed the comforting illusion that they would always be strong and hard.

In addition, like most people, I miss various vanished dreams and opportunities, chances, forks in the road of life, that will never come again. In my most quiet, private moments, it's the eternal question of What if I had done this or that differently? that causes me the most anguish. For me, at least, the pain of the loss of a breast pales in comparison.

And my husband's attitude when I faced losing a breast? I knew that all that would matter to David, all that ever could matter to him, was whether or not I stayed alive. This last realization was a profound reaffirmation of his love, and there is no other result of my illness that has offered me more comfort and reassurance.

## Fear and Progress

*[There are two doctors mentioned in this section. Dr. Brew is the surgeon who performed my mastectomy, and Dr. Baumgartner is my primary care physician.]*

Even after I had survived the surgery itself, even after a year, and then two, and then three whole years had passed with no recurrence of the disease for me, I found that I was afraid, at least on some level. I feared that no matter how strong or health conscious or upbeat I might be, cancer could come creeping again.

Most of the time, my fear was rather slight, something I could shove to the back of my mind. It became a sort of intermittent static, only occasionally distracting. There never seemed to be much point in talking about it, even to David. For what could he have said to reassure me? I knew that he was afraid, too, afraid that Death might change its mind and come back to claim me after all.

Thus David and I had a largely unspoken agreement that we would remain as upbeat and as busy as we could, getting on with our shared and separate lives, acting as though we were confident of decades more together. We almost never used actual words to articulate our worry to one another. An extra hug or kiss in the course of the day, a particularly tender caress as we lay together in bed—those could speak volumes.

In the late summer of 2003, the required round of medical examinations showed me free of cancer after five whole years. Dr. Brew congratulated me and told me that of course I should continue getting yearly physical exams from Dr. Baumgartner and yearly mammograms, but that I no longer needed to come to her for checkups. I hugged her goodbye with tears in my eyes, feeling again a great wash of gratitude for all her excellent care.

Is every vestige of my fear of future cancer now gone? No, it isn't. To feel no more fear at all would be illogical. But between that last examination by Dr. Brew and now, the intermittent static has quieted considerably.

Now I feel that having a mastectomy did much more than merely postpone my death. With infinite gratitude to Dr. Brew and all the others, I feel that I was given a second chance at life.

## Aging, Accepting, and Appreciating

Gray hair, wrinkles, age spots, crooked and darkening teeth, sagging body contours, spider veins—most women in our society see these as horrors that must be held at bay for as long as possible, no matter what the cost.

Am I immune from such concerns? Of course not. I dyed my unexciting, light brown hair varying shades of blond, red-blond, and red for more than a dozen years. Over twenty years ago, I had some crooked teeth straightened. Later on, I had my teeth bleached. Every couple of months, I go to a wonderful aesthetician for a facial and a micro-dermabrasion treatment. Sometime in the near future, I hope to have sclerotherapy treatments (multi-site injections) for some unsightly spider veins and new varicose veins which have appeared on my legs. And I'm now trying to shape up and firm up as much as I can with diet and exercise.

But there are limits to how far I'll go to try to maintain a youthful appearance. In part, this attitude is due to my wish to emulate other women whom I admire. A former weight training student of mine, a woman in her seventies with a stunning cap of pure white hair, was one of my primary models of how to grow old gracefully. Also, after careful observation of many women closer to my own age who had made the bold decision to relax and go with the gray, I decided that most of them looked not old, but serene and self-confident. That was a look I longed for.

Thus I quit coloring my hair just before I had my mastectomy, figuring that the dye was not something I needed to subject my skin to any longer. A few months later, I was rewarded with the delightful comment from a male acquaintance that the new color—light brown with some gray, especially in the front and on the top—had a "soft ease" about it.

Now I really love both my short, simple hairstyle and my hair's natural color.

For me, it had finally come down to a matter of acceptance, the acceptance of the reality of being middle-aged. Today I count my new, calmer attitude toward aging as one of the most significant benefits of having survived cancer. After my mastectomy, I was simply glad to be alive. After that, each new birthday felt like a wonderful gift. My dread of aging was vaporized. Along with the dread went most of my personal vanity and concern about looking as young as possible.

After my cancer, I realized that I was tired of trying so hard to look young, tired of my old preoccupation with my appearance. There were so many other, better avenues for my energies! The pursuit of continued and better health had to be my number one priority. After that, I had to make sure my family and friends knew how much I loved and appreciated them. I also saw that the multiple areas of my working life needed some serious attention, some sorting and prioritizing.

Then again, perhaps my cancer experience merely accelerated a process of acceptance that had been set into motion some time before, shortly after I passed 50—a milestone which often seems to mark a turning point in people's lives, be they men or women. On the other side of that milestone, there is often a new landscape of calm and purpose.

I've learned that it's not uncommon for those of 50 and beyond to seek out new horizons—learning, creating, traveling, relating to others in new ways—even while they peacefully accept the demise of old dreams and ambitions that they finally recognize will never be fulfilled. For those lucky enough to experience it, it's a profoundly joyful, liberating, and even exciting process.

From talking to many others, as well as from my own experience, I've learned that surviving a serious accident or illness greatly accelerates this normal progression. Such an experience shows you what's really important in life. It allows you to focus in a way you may never have dreamed possible prior to that life altering event.

That's partly because recovery forces you to slow down, to alter or even suspend your normal daily routine, perhaps for a long period of time. In the newly quiet spaces, you can hear your innermost voices. Listen well to them, for they are very wise. Those voices can urge you to let go of many an old vanity or ambition. They can soothe old hurts, telling you to let go and forgive. They can point the way toward some new path that you should take: professionally, personally, or both.

Last but scarcely least, survival teaches you a new appreciation of all the good things in life: love of family and friends, little daily pleasures, and the beauty that surrounds us but which we all too often ignore. I was never blind to such things, but my cancer brought all of them into much sharper focus.

At times, now, I stand amazed at how much joy even very little things can bring me: the rich brown of my morning tea in its cobalt cup, the tang of fresh blueberries with my cereal, the soothing sounds of the classical music that accompanies my writing, the scent of welcome rain on the parched Colorado landscape, the sight of two frisky squirrels playing tag around the trunk of a tree.

It sometimes feels as though I was ill and then reborn. When I awoke, I saw the world with new eyes, the appreciative, eager eyes of a child. May those fresh eyes never grow dull again!

# 15.

# Moment by Painful Moment, I Am Learning

## BY FAY OCTAVIA ELLIOTT

*After a thirty year corporate career, Fay is currently pursuing a masters in divinity degree full time. She plans to become an interfaith hospice chaplain. FayElliott@FullyAwakeInc.com.*

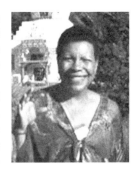

I have never called myself a breast cancer survivor. It has the sound of being a victim of breast cancer. From the moment I was diagnosed, I was determined that my life would be the better for it on the other end. I believe ultimately this mindset has benefited me in ways I am only beginning to understand.

My life shattered Thanksgiving weekend 1995. My husband Michael and I went shopping for furniture for our living room. One minute we were sitting at a traffic light and the next minute, I had a huge headache, and Michael was slumped over in his seat with blood dripping from his nose. It would be days before I returned home from the hospital, and Michael would only return once many months later. Eventually they told me that Michael had pulled out into the intersection before the light changed, and we had been hit on the driver's side of the car by a tractor trailer truck.

The accident was the beginning of an eighteen month ordeal for Michael and a many years ordeal for me. He had a traumatic brain injury and was in a coma for over six months. Then, when he was conscious, he could not talk or move. After eighteen months (with my help) he was able to request to be taken off life support. He died in March 1997.

They sent me home from the hospital two days after the accident and told me I could go back to work. I had been meditating for a few years by then and could tell something was wrong with my brain. I was attention deficit and my mind was more chaotic when I sat down to meditate than I would have expected even given my emotional trauma with Michael's injuries. I was eventually diagnosed with a mild traumatic brain injury. My IQ scores had dropped into a very low range, and I could not focus on anything. I also could not recall common expressions and could barely think at all when my brain was tired. Before the accident, I was a management consultant in a "big six" accounting firm. After the accident I could barely function in any capacity, let alone do work at the level required by my firm.

On Thanksgiving weekend two years after the accident, I felt a pain in my right breast and when I touched it, I felt a lump. Eventually the lump was diagnosed as breast cancer.

I made every attempt to save the breast initially. There were several lumpectomies and chemotherapy. Then we discovered a cluster of calcium deposits. These deposits were a second completely different cancer in the same breast. The second cancer had been forming for awhile. Four years earlier, I had a stereotactic biopsy in the same area because there were calcium deposits there. At that time no malignancy was found. This time when they found cells that they were malignant, I had a mastectomy and breast replacement surgery in December 1998.

From the moment my cancer was diagnosed, I went into the same mindset that I used when solving a problem in my profession. I researched cancer treatments and alternative treatments. Based on the information at hand, mastectomy, chemotherapy and radiation therapy were the conventional treatments that were available. There did not seem to be any alternative treatments that had any research to support them. It did seem that Chinese herbal medicine could mitigate some of the toxic effects of chemotherapy. I started interviewing oncologists to see what options they would offer me and to find one that would work with alternative medicine alongside the conventional therapy. First I found a Chinese herbalist, and she gave me a referral to another of her client's oncologist. He was very likable and willing to work with a patient using alternative approaches, too.

At the time of the cancer diagnosis, I was exhausted from years of "workaholism," my brain injury from the accident, and the strain of Michael's long ordeal. I decided I wanted to be in better shape after my cancer experience than I was going in. The first thing I did was take a medical leave of absence so I could rest and recover without distractions. I was fortunate enough to have long-term disability coverage and was able to stop working for almost a year which I really needed. Then I started walking two miles every day, practicing yoga and eating an all-vegetarian diet. I continued my research and found a doctor who had some success with cancer remission using healing meditation and visualization exercises. I met with one of his counselors, and he taught me the meditation techniques.

Part of the meditation process was a visualization to talk with the cancer cells and see why they were in your body. I was not really surprised when they told me that I wanted to die. My life was so stressful. I traveled all the time and was never home with my husband. When we were together, we were both strained by my coming and going and found it difficult to really connect. There was no time in my life for socializing, friends, family or just plain fun. I lived on airplanes and in hotel rooms. In a hypnotherapy session, we discovered that the little girl in me was very mad because she said we never had time to play.

When I was home recovering from the cancer, my friends all said, "You do too much." No one knew anyone as busy as I seemed to be even not working and being on chemo. The other thing my friends all said to me is that "You are always taking care of other people, but don't seem to take time for yourself." Overdoing and care taking certainly have been a pattern of mine my whole adult life. I believe my breast cancer was affected by taking hormone replacement therapy for early onset menopause. However, I suspect that overdoing, care taking and lack of self-care may be primary contributing factors to lowering my immune function and causing me to be more susceptible to breast cancer.

While I was on chemotherapy, I started having severe anxiety attacks caused by the drugs. The medications they tried to alleviate them only seemed to exaggerate them. My meditation practice helped me once again. What I discovered as I sat with the anxiety was that my attempts to push it away only made it escalate. My capacity to sit with the anxious feelings and just let the experience be what it was eventually caused the anxiety to fade away. Again, without my meditation practice, I don't think I would have so quickly recognized signs of depression when they arrived or sought help. I used medications for a short while but ultimately found my mindfulness meditation practice was more beneficial.

While on leave, I studied hypnotherapy and mindfulness-based stress reduction. In the years since that experience, I returned to my profession as a consultant and ultimately decided that I wanted to spend the second half of my life giving back and doing something of more value to the world. It seemed that my experience with Michael's death and my own cancer were preparation for something. Then I went through a similar experience with my mother's death in 2005. I knew I had valuable experience to share with others after facing the possibility of my own death and the death of my dearest loved ones. In March 2008, I started volunteering with a hospice. When I found out you needed a master of divinity degree to become a hospice chaplain, I enrolled in a contemplative religious education program.

After the car accident, it felt that my life was completely out of my control. The only thing I had control over was my response. So moment by painful moment, grounded in my mindfulness practice, I responded to each situation as it occurred. At one point, my husband's social worker referred me to a therapist because she was concerned about me. I later learned her concern was that I was too calm. Only after she attended a meditation retreat with me did she apologize and tell me she understood why I was handling the situation the way I did. She realized that I was not in denial about what was happening but that my meditation practice gave me the mental capacity to be calm in the midst of an emotionally stormy situation.

My meditation teacher often spoke about his mentor, Gandhi. Gandhi would say, "I love storms." He said Gandhi was at his best when the opposition was strongest. Over time, I have experienced that I am at my best when pitted against the most difficult situations. It is almost as if my mind works best when challenged. Certainly I thought that nothing would ever be as challenging as the situation I experienced while my husband was dying. In retrospect, perhaps because I was prepared to face challenges from that experience, my own cancer experience was not nearly as difficult to face as it would have been.

When I was retested five years after the accident, my IQ scores were in the above average range and most of my mental functioning had returned. Even today, my brain still shuts down when it gets tired, but in general, I seem to think better than I did before the accident. The neuro-psychologists were very surprised because most recovery happens early, and I continued to recover over time. I continued my meditation and other visualization practices throughout those years. One doctor said that most patients with brain injuries do not have the concentration needed to practice meditation. Because I had meditation experience before the accident, I was able to use it to restore and in some ways improve my brain's functioning. The benefits of my mindfulness meditation practice continue even today as you will see.

In 2009, I had a headache that lasted ten weeks and was exhausted all the time. When I was twenty, I had an autoimmune disease called sarcoidosis which affected my lungs and my energy level. The doctors said it can be caused by stress. At that time, I was both working and going to school full-time. Thirty years later, I am a lot older and going to school full-time and working half-time. It seems some lessons are never learned. Perhaps from stress again, that illness is reoccurring in a chronic form. One doctor said the headaches seem to be related to the head injury and chemotherapy affects on my brain.

I reached a very low point and thought that perhaps dying would be easier than facing being sick and tired for the rest my life. Then I had a moment of realizing that just because my body was in pain and struggling; it didn't mean that my mind needed to be in pain and struggling. I made a decision to work with my mindfulness meditation practice even more. I knew about lots of people who were happy and joyful despite much worse physical conditions. Why couldn't it be true for me too? I deepened my mindfulness practice, stopped my part-time work and volunteer activities and continued with just my full-time studies. I even occasionally go to the movies and video arcade with some of the other students who are less than half my age.

A few weeks ago, I was diagnosed with a reoccurrence of breast cancer. It appears that some breast tissue from the original site had migrated to a muscle under my arm. After the tumor was removed, the doctor told me that if the tumor has metastasized, there might be very little they could do for me and if not, my situation was very curable with conventional therapies. The most surprising thing was my response. Right then I knew that whichever way it went, I was prepared to work with it. If I were dying, then I would die well. My mind was clear and ready to work with the situation. On the other hand, if the prognosis was good, I would have to face chemotherapy and radiation therapy. On some level, the thought of going through cancer treatment again was enough to make me think death would be preferable. That night while I was still in the hospital, I decided I could face the treatments and whatever else I might experience one moment at a time. Once again, I realized that my mind did not have to be high-jacked by my experience. Just as I chose my response those many years ago after the car accident, I could choose my response now. My faithful mindfulness practice still provides me with the tools to work with my situation moment by moment.

The subsequent PET scan shows no evidence of metastases or residual activity. Still my oncologist advised that I should undergo a round of chemotherapy and radiation therapy as a precautionary measure. I am committed once again to being in better condition at the end than I am now. I plan to work with a nutritionist that specializes in working with cancer patients and a Chinese herbalist that specializes in working with women's issues. Both are highly recommended, and I feel certain they will make a big difference in how I feel through the process. Of course, my mind is one of the most powerful tools of all and my mindfulness practice will continue to support my well-being.

Remembering my experience with chemotherapy the last time, I know that I will have to conserve my energy more and more as I get nearer to the end of the treatment. So, while I plan to continue my studies full-time, I will cut back to the minimum number of credits. In the meanwhile, for my chaplaincy project next semester, I plan to facilitate a healing meditation group for people with cancer and chronic illness and will offer a mindfulness-based stress reduction group for students on campus dealing with stress. Along with another woman who also has had breast cancer twice, we are designing a four-stage program for women with breast cancer. The program will educate a woman about the stage she currently finds herself in and provide tools and support for navigating through that stage, i.e., hearing a new diagnosis, being in treatment, recovering from treatment, and living life after cancer.

I imagine you are wondering when I will slow down. I plan to spend the rest of the summer resting and (indeed) will play as well. I am learning a lot about self-care from my training and have lots of good friends in my life now who take care of me and remind me to take care of myself.

When I was at my lowest point the first time I had cancer and more recently when diagnosed with chronic sarcoidosis and chronic headaches, I thought that dying might be easier than facing life as it is. I have learned from working with my own mind that I can face life as it is joyfully and peacefully even when my body isn't working and my life seems out of control. I know (too) that facing my husband's and mother's deaths and my own illnesses gives me awesome credibility for working with people and their families experiencing sickness and death. They know that I have walked in their shoes and while our experiences may be nothing alike, my heart is open, my compassion deep, and my resolve to stick with them through the storms and the fire is unflinching.

Both times I faced breast cancer, I had to acknowledge how I had failed to take care of myself. Breast cancer has twice given me an opportunity to refocus on my healing and wholeness. Maybe you can "teach an old dog new tricks." This time breast cancer has also given me a new sense of commitment to living my life as full out as I can at every moment and taking exquisite care of myself while still being of the greatest possible benefit to others. This is what it means to me to be a breast cancer thriver.

# 16.
# A Breast of Wisdom—
# What About Healing?

## BY RAYWYN M. ERICKSON

*Raywyn M. Erickson is gifted with unique abilities allowing her to empower others by gently helping them connect with and understand their feeling nature. She is the author of 'The Rainbow Highway', a collection of tools, theories and techniques to help us understand being human and our life purpose. Through her books, teachings and consultations she invites people to look within for their unique key-ways to success. Raywyn M Erickson, RScP: Wholistic Education Consultant, A\*S\*K\* CENTRE for SUCCESS! www.ask4success.com / raywyme@shaw.ca*

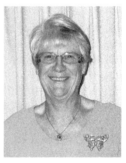

It was Summer 2008 when I discovered a dimple on my left breast as I applied my deodorant one morning. I was shocked yet calm at the same time, remembering a friend sharing her story with me many years ago. It took me a few weeks to find a woman doctor who examined me and sent me for the usual mammograms which I'd had previously a long time ago. It didn't make any sense to focus on looking for lumps believing the universal law, that what you pay attention to, you get to experience.

Two mammograms, two bilateral breast MRI's and ultrasound biopsies later they told me it would take 7 to 10 days for my doctor to receive the report. I left the hospital at 3:20 pm and early the next morning, before opening time, a surgeon's office called me to come in immediately. While I sat in the surgeon's office she read the report saying "We don't like this" and "You know what that means" as she circled words on the report. She talked about the removal surgery, and the plastic surgeon coming to do reconstructive surgery at the same time on the left and possibly the right breast. She spoke of wigs, chemotherapy and radiation but never did she mention the "C" word. There were eight tumors found in my breasts, three in my lymph glands, and the two larger ones on my left breast tested positive "malignant". At this stage, I refused more biopsies to damage my breasts, thereby creating more physical healing for the body to recover as I was aware all the intervention would need to heal at some time.

The surgeon left me alone in the room to copy the report for me and I heard my inner voice calling out "What about healing?" I sat there calm but stunned yet I knew to listen to my inner voice "Cancer is not the problem, cancer is the cure!" Cure for what, I wondered? "Consciousness" was the reply. Upon the surgeon's return I asked "What about healing?" to which she replied "We'll talk about that later." I thought, "I don't think so" and I left her office on a quest... I knew this was my "calling".

I met my finance' Ian outside and burst into tears, feeling overwhelmed and angry. He was very supportive though scared in his own way, and he reassured me that whatever I needed to do to get this out of my body he would be there for me. We had lots of heart warming discussions which has brought us closer together. He was very encouraging and often commented on my courage to walk this path. This then meant putting my money where my mouth was and walking my talk by putting into practice what I believed was right for me about the diagnosis.

Fortunately, the surgeon was going on three weeks vacation, and then my doctor was going on three weeks vacation so that gave me six weeks leeway—a grace period so to speak.—Next morning I canceled my appointment and told the receptionist I was not going for the surgery—I was going on a healing journey. I phoned my doctor who was very understanding and supportive and asked me to keep the lines of communication open. My Doctor said, "If she needed surgery she'd go to her surgeon as she was the best person to do it. This was a vote of confidence if I chose to change my mind—no doesn't mean never.

I immediately got on the phone to the people who had the information I needed and began my journey within to discover the emotional traumas and hurts, or old resentments I had buried or nursed. I explored the time lines and traced the journey back to the episodes in my life that left me feeling hurt, and threatened my sense of self and safety. It was truly amazing and became so clear as I progressed. I remembered incidents during my developing years and things I'd filed away in my belief system, true or false, there they were like seeds waiting for the right time to grow. (I could write a book about these, but that's another story.)

A big discovery for me was both the type of comments and the lack of comments from friends and family members as I shared my journey with them. It brought up their own fears, their fear of losing me, and so it became about them. That was a shocking realization for me when I didn't receive the support that I needed from them—a big wake-up call for sure!

Even though I'd hoped it wasn't true, I had a knowing that it was, and all my previous thoughts came racing into my mind trying to make sense and validate this experience. I had reached a point in my life where I was reaping the rewards of my quest which began in 1985 when my husband had a heart attack, and I learned to help him through his journey until he made his transition in February 1992. I had discovered a lot and was sharing this information to help others and now dealing with my own human frailties was to be a catalyst for more effective communication skills.

None of my immediate family history revealed breast cancer, especially on my mother's side. I'd never been pregnant and I knew bits and pieces of the myths and facts floating around the world. I'd traveled from New Zealand to Great Britain to meet all my relatives in England, Scotland and Wales in the 1960's. I'd traveled around Europe and Scandinavia to meet my grandparents relatives and friends. I'd lived in South Africa in the 1970's and finally heeded my childhood calling (a story I'd written when I was about eight years old, titled 'When I grow up I will live in Canada'). I'd always wanted to be a teacher, a nurse or a police woman but I was too young, so off I went to see the world.

In 1976 I came to Canada, met my husband in 1977, married in 1978 and I am still here over 30 years later. I bless him for allowing me to stay in one place and get to know myself. I became a teacher—a wholistic educator—facilitating groups to help people to understand their stress and transform fear into personal freedom. People were having healing experiences and amazing results from the information I shared—so living my heart's desire. I also became a writer with my first book, *"Living Choices: Key-ways to meet the challenge of change".* While writing this book, I met Doctor Nelie Johnson, who was promoting *"taking the fear out of breast cancer"* and she described the biological and scientific proof for understanding the way the body works. It was awesome. It made everything make sense and I was so excited.

I wanted to share my beliefs around illness and disease and paying attention to our thoughts, feelings and core beliefs. I supported a friend through chemotherapy in 2007 and I also knew two women who underwent different surgeries. I spoke to them and also two women who refused surgery and are still living today. I even met strangers who shared their stories giving me encouragement and support.

I was shocked when the surgeon's office called me two months later to come in for an update. She listened to me talk about what I was doing, and then said "Now you listen to me!" I knew from the change of her voice and attitude she didn't know what I was talking about. She then proceeded to tell me the facts and figures from the last ten years and the billions of dollars spent on breast cancer research. She told me to talk to the oncologist for more up-to-date details which I did. I had the feeling she was trying to push me into surgery and the oncologist was another medical authority for me to deal with. But that's another story. He confirmed that my type of cancer, estrogen fed, was treatable after chemotherapy and radiation with Tamoxofin tablets. He informed me they don't know the cause, they don't have a cure and there are no guarantees and asked, "Now why wouldn't I consent to the surgery?" to which I replied "Why would I?—There are people healing themselves." He wasn't happy with my reply and left the office saying, if I needed to talk to him further, I could do so through the surgeon.

Imagine my feelings when I heard on the local radio news shortly after that the Fraser Valley Health Authority had a mandate to operate on everyone diagnosed with breast cancer within three weeks, and they'd met their mandate. To them, that was a good thing, but for me you can imagine how that kind of thinking feeds the fear. New and larger cancer treatment hospitals are opening all over the place—it is big business.

I had learned and believe that stress is a precursor; a symptom to wake us up prior to any illness. I used to think stress was my middle name and thought it was normal to feel fearful and anxious. I then learned tapping techniques to release the energy like EFT (Emotional Freedom Technique) and the Dynamind Process which gave me permission to experience and express negative thoughts and feelings. I learned about food combining and the yeast connection—something I had struggled with most of my life. There are also chemical reactions from household products, toiletries and cosmetics which affect our nervous systems. I heard about the pH balance of water and how we need more oxygen in our bodies and how cancer cells love sugar, acidic environments—another issue I had most of my life. I also know that feelings are the universal language of the Soul vibrating, pulsating, and communicating through the cells in our body to let us know where we are at in this moment. I learned about the thyroid connection and how stress compromised my immune system and much, much more. I wish I had learned about these things in school—about the body systems, center point systems, meridians and connectedness. I was afraid of my own blood, my own shadow, never mind my light.

Now I had to question "What does self-healing mean to me?" The quest began again. My first spiritual awakening as a result of doing the 12-step program of Al-Anon in 1988 was—Acceptance—I felt the Gift of Receiving—and now I was being called to this in a new way. Acceptance—doesn't mean liking it—it is what it is, learn to work with it on life's terms. I learned we must feel it to heal it, release old hurts and resentments blocking the energy flow and allowing the lymph glands to do their work. I learned physical exercises and Yoga helping the mind/body to let go, releasing blocks in the energy flowing through my systems. I had Louise Hay's book *"You Can Heal Your Life"* which has been like a bible to me since 1987. *"Feelings Buried Alive Never Die..."* (Karol Kuhn-Truman) are two books that helped me tremendously along the way.

I discovered you can't kill energy; it just shifts vibrations and changes form.

I knew I was avoiding the next level of my Life—to learn about vibrations and energy work and go beyond the known. I studied Ayurveda (Magical Mind—Magical Body by Deepak Chopra and many other books and his philosophy for life) and met a woman I knew 20 years ago, Jaisri Lambert who was now a qualified Ayurvedic consultant so I began the Ayurvedic self-healing program with herbs to cleanse and stimulate the body systems—back to balance and wholeness—something I'd been curious about for years, the whole body/mind-emotional/spiritual connection. She told me "Absence of illness is not the signature of wellness!" Now I was getting really excited to learn more.

I attended classes I'd previously been interested but only dabbled in, stopping when my current love relationship started and I moved to Surrey in 1993 to study Life Skills. I began relearning meditation, visualization, affirmations and self honesty at new levels. I gave myself more mental, emotional, physical, and spiritual value and credibility and amazing things have occurred beyond my wildest imagination. I shared and gave back what I had learned, helping others to understand themselves. I started volunteering again, sharing with women in transition with amazing results. It was as if something in me had changed and it was no longer like speaking a foreign language. The women were eager to learn this stuff because now it makes more sense to them. "A miracle is a heartfelt shift in perception"—Pinocchio.

I was invited to be the keynote guest speaker at a graduation because I'd been the most inspirational teacher they had during their program. This was a miracle to me and I knew the healing was happening because people were coming back into my life since I'd been doing my forgiveness work—it was truly remarkable!

People now comment on how peaceful and calming my energy is and they love to be in my company. I feel better now than I did most of my life and that feels great! I am learning by sharing and what used to be very difficult to share is much easier as a sense of maturity and wisdom prevails.

In conclusion, I was teaching "You don't have to be sick to get better"—I never felt sick before, during or after my diagnosis. I have had to face being wrong and right... (And that was scary). If I had the ability to heal myself what else would be required of me? My life changed for the better because I realized I can't keep putting off living my dream, I must live it daily.. Discovering the power within, in other words my creative intelligence, genius, spirituality and self, means that I have a divine connection with my inner being.

What an amazing journey it is!

*I'd like to take this opportunity to acknowledge some of the people who shared their gifts and wisdom with me on this amazing healing journey, and if I missed anyone, you know who you are, and please accept my blessings.*

*Ian H. Engledow-Currie who is sharing this amazing journey with me daily. Cathrine Levan, Karin Jander, Debra Taylor, Janan Thomas, Carla Muth, Joan Bingham, Jessie Loraine English, Jeanie Mackie, Moreah Vandevalde, April Farrall, Suzanne Robinson, Monique MacDonald, Jan Janzen, Judy LeBeau-Harris, Zosia Ettenberg, Eleanor Wells and the Valley Women's Network, Susan D'Agastino, Kala H. Kos, Margaret O'Brien, Kelsey Cameron, Dr. Nelie Johnson, Dr. Caroline Markolin, German New Medicine, Dr.Sanjay Mohan Ram and the team at Mountain Wellness Centre, Dr. Teresa Clarke and the team at Inspire Health—Integrative Cancer/Health Care, plus Evie (Norma) Mahoney for editing this project, and Beverly Vote for inviting me to get this typed—a big thank you!*

BreastCancerWellness.org

# 17.

# A Huge Step in My Recovery

## BY ANNE ERICSON

*Anne Ericson is 67 years old. In 1995 she was reacquainted with a high school friend, Eric Ericson, the love of her life. They have been married for 14 wonderful years. Together they have five sons, and three grandchildren. Anne and Eric enjoy dancing to the 50's and 60's music that they grew up with. They love traveling to countries such as China, France, Italy and many places in the US. They enjoy their log home in the country, working in their flowers and garden, entertaining friends and driving their 2006 Corvette. Anne has no intention of retiring anytime soon. Anne Ericson CMF, CFm, annee@americanbreastcare.com*

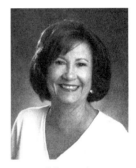

I am a 37 year breast cancer thriver. My healing journey began in early October 1973, a couple weeks before my 30th birthday. At the end of a busy day, I was taking a nice warm bath and I felt a lump in my right breast about the size of the tip of my little finger. It was in the upper outer quadrant. I've learned over the years this is the general area 50% of lumps are located. I was not one to do self breast exams, not at my age. I did not feel any thing in my left breast. My first thoughts were, "Don't panic, I'm sure it is nothing and it will be gone tomorrow."

I was a stay at home mom with two boys. Kenny, my eleven year old, was into year round sports and Jeff, my six year old, was into everything. My life was one busy whirl wind. Team mother, room mother, PTA member, and any thing my boys volunteered me to do. I didn't mention I was married, not the greatest marriage in the world. We stayed together because it was the right thing to do for the boys.

There was another situation going on at that time, my 52 year old dad had been diagnosed with lung cancer. Yes, he was a heavy smoker. My mother was not handling my dad's illness very well. I was an only child, thus I was the only one there for my mother and dad. My plate was full to the brim. I did not have time to be having problems with my breast or anything else for that matter.

After a couple days of not mentioning this to anyone, the lump was still there with no change. I vaguely mentioned this to my mother while waiting for my dad to take another cobalt treatment. Well needless to say, that very afternoon I had a appointment with dad's doctor who was aware of my mother's concern. To put it mildly, she was frantic. My doctor did not seem to be alarmed, but suggested I see a surgeon. And the doctor who specialized in breast surgery was not concerned either but suggested having a biopsy. His suggestion was as much to put my mother's mind at ease. In those days, a biopsy meant a two day stay in the hospital. We scheduled the surgery for a few weeks later because of two important upcoming birthdays to celebrate. My oldest son's 12th birthday was October 16 and my 30th birthday was October 20. My hopes were that just maybe the lump would go away during this time.

I remember driving to the old St. Thomas Hospital in Nash for the scheduled operation for the biopsy in November and thinking what a waste of time even though the lump hadn't gone away. I nearly backed out but knowing what my mother's reaction would be, I checked into the hospital. My surgery was scheduled the next morning. Oh well, I thought, not a big deal.

When I was waking up the following afternoon after the surgery, I caught a glimpse of my aunt Jean, my cousin Juan, and half dozen other friends and relatives I had not seen in a while. I thought they must not have anything better to do and I went back to sleep. As I began to come back to reality and my brain kicked in, I began to realize something wasn't exactly right.

The next thing I remember my surgeon came in and broke the news that the lump had shown some activity. In other words I had cancer in my breast. He had already scheduled me to go back into surgery the next day for a radical mastectomy.

Well, I've heard of the black hole, or the pit, but I had not had that experience until then. The only way to describe the black hole is that you are there alone. I'm sure I was given something to make me rest because I don't remember anything until the next morning before I went into surgery. The days that followed were not too painful, I just couldn't lift my arm due to the lymph nodes that were removed. One day a lady came into my room to give me some information and to show me some exercises to do for my arm. She was from Reach to Recovery, a volunteer program made up of women who were breast cancer survivors. All I could think of was ,"Yeah right, I bet she didn't have the same surgery I've had, or else she couldn't use her arm." She told me to start doing my exercises as soon as my doctor said I could, they would help get my physical strength back. She left me a bra and a puff to wear when I felt like it. The same day the doctor gave me the good news that no lymph nodes were affected and that my prognosis looked good.

The next day was NOT a good day, it was the day my bandages were removed. As soon as the nurse left I went to the mirror for the viewing. Well, it was not a pretty sight, no nipple, not even a little bump. The scar went half way across my chest and under my arm with a whole big enough for a tennis ball. All I could do was sit down and cry. I cried long and hard and uncontrollably. While I was crying I felt a very light touch on my shoulder. I didn't look up, but I could see her white nurses shoes. I never knew who she was but that gentle touch helped to quiet my tears and my anguish. Somehow this unselfish act of compassion gave me the strength I needed which became the first major step to my recovery and my journey.

The next thing I did, after I wiped away the tears, was to reach for the bra and puff the lady from Reach to Recovery had left me. I put on some makeup, put on my bra and puff, and my new gown and matching robe, it was blue, and went for a walk. The old hospitals had long halls, so I walked all the way down to the other end of the hospital. Without realizing it, I must have wandered into the men's section. I was almost at the end when I heard a whistle, not looking in that direction, I thought could that whistle be for me? Well, I claimed it anyway, turned and started back to my room, I held my head up and my shoulders back as well as I could, went back to my room and decided right then and there, I was still the young lady as the day I checked myself into the hospital. I could get a whistle then and I could get one now. That was the second huge step towards my recovery and my journey.

Six months to the day, May 9th, 1974, my dad died from lung cancer.

Soon after, I wanted to do something to help women going through breast surgery. I became a volunteer for Reach to Recovery. I was the youngest volunteer in the Davidson County Unit. I was active with this organization for ten years. I loved making my visits and doing what I could to help a lady feel better and give her some encouragement. Helping women was another huge step in my recovery and my journey.

In 1978, I was divorced from Tom. It really had nothing to do with my surgery. I needed to move on.

In 1983, my mother passed from cancer. It was another black hole again.

I went to work at a bank in Nash. During that time, I began to meet more people in the breast care business. I did some public speaking about my experience and Reach to Recovery. In 1985, my youngest son, Jeff, started college. A friend in Atlanta Georgia called to tell me about an ad she had read in the Atlanta newspaper. It was for a sales representative for a company that manufactured silicone breast prostheses. I was familiar with the company. I called and got a interview in Atlanta for the next day. I had never driven more than 100 miles outside of Nash alone but I headed out to Atlanta. I had two interviews and I was hired. I had never flown before and was mortified but the first flight for my job was incredible. I had seven, yes that's seven states in my territory: Tennessee, Virginia, North Carolina, South Carolina, Georgia, Alabama, and Mississippi. This company was serious about serving the prosthetic needs of women facing breast cancer. Twenty five years later, I am the Breast Care Specialist for American Breast Care, working for the same wonderful people I started with. I have four states now.

I have had the pleasure of meeting and working with women all over the southeast. I train new fitters, show new products to my accounts, and have the opportunity of during promotions to work and fit our customers. My goal and mission, as is my company's, is helping women look and feel better about themselves after breast surgery. It gives me great joy to see a woman's face light up and see her walk out of the fitting room wearing her new pretty bra with a soft and natural prostheses.

In 1996, I married the love of my life, Eric. He is supportive of my career and knows how much I love my work. He has never made me feel less of a woman because of my surgery. He is a wonderful man and I am very blessed to have him in my life. He's handsome, too!

I'll celebrate my 67th birthday on October 20. I've been a Survivor and Thriver over half of my life. I can truly say I have no regrets. I believe things happen for a reason. I believe we have choices to turn a bad situation into a positive one. I believe our attitudes about ourselves make a difference in our recovery. I never wanted to hide the fact I had a mastectomy.

I would like to thank my mother for pushing me to have the biopsy, I may have waited too late otherwise. My two sons for knowing their mother is a survivor and a thriver and for being supportive. Thanks to my husband, Eric, for being the loving man he is and my two stepsons and three grandchildren for loving me as I am. Thanks to my best friend,

Judy, who encouraged me every day to do my exercises for my arm. And thanks to the two mystery people, the nurse and the whistler. I never had a chance to thank them for giving me strength, courage and hope. And to American Breast Care, my wonderful company that keeps manufacturing the most innovative, high-quality products for the women we serve.

# 18.

# Choice

## BY NEDRA FILLMER

*Nedra Fillmer is a 13 year Breast Cancer Thriver. She and her husband, Roger, have been married for 35 years and are the parents of two sons. Since she recently retired her days are now spent with her husband, friends and doing the things that she loves, like quilting, cooking, traveling and enjoying her new home. fillmernedra@yahoo.com*

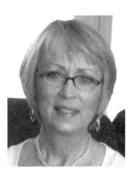

When given a choice are we willing to step out there and grasp it? Where did cancer fit into my choices? When I was diagnosed with cancer the word choice took on a whole new meaning. Did I have a choice? Was it something I did or did not do? I believe every woman diagnosed with breast cancer will endure her own personal turmoil until she makes her peace with the things she has no control over. I felt that my body had betrayed me and I struggled for years to find my "happy" place again. Once I realized that I had a choice; cancer could become my life or just be a part of my past. It is not an easy journey but it is a journey worth traveling.

I was diagnosed with breast cancer at 42 years old. I had found a large lump by accident and a biopsy was performed on a simple cyst—or so they said—until it returned from pathology. It then had officially become cancer and I was scheduled for a mastectomy. At that time, my husband and I had one child in college and one in high school and our lives were very busy. My husband, Roger, was an officer in the National Guard and worked for the Federal Aviation Administration. Between the two, this kept him out of town often and I worked full time in the administration office at school. Just like anyone diagnosed with cancer, your life becomes a whirl wind of doctor appointments. I was very fortunate that my mother was available to help take me back and forth for treatments. Life then for the next five years was like most breast cancer survivors, from one doctor to the next. I remember the feeling of fear when I hit my five year mark—suddenly no one would be "watching" over me, and how would I know if the cancer returned? Over the course of several years I had a multitude of health problems, or things that were out of my control... or was I just being overly cautious to the point that my body was reacting to my fear?

Who is to say, but today I try to apply this analogy to my life: As I go through life, I have a "choice" and there are situations which I encounter and refer to as "rocks" along the road. My choices are to either pick that rock up and carry it with me or leave it beside life's road. Sometimes I might carry the rock for a while but when it is time, I have to let the rock go. I could not change the fact that cancer entered my life but I could change how it affected my life and my future.

Today I try not to ever turn down an opportunity to enrich my life. That often means stepping beyond my comfort zone into unknown territory. My husband and I have both taken an early retirement and we recently returned from a trip to South Africa, along with a trip to Colorado with our ATV's not something I ever felt I would ever do. For years, I "played it safe" staying in a routine only doing or going to the places where I knew the outcomes. But I have realized that I only truly found my "happy" place by choosing to step out and trying new and exciting things. You to have a choice to learn from your experiences, step out on faith and GROW through this portion of your life into a better phase of life. Only you can make the choice to thrive instead of just survive.

# 19.
# How to Help Your Wife Thrive

## BY PETER FLIERL

*Peter J. Flierl, MSW is the author of the award winning book, "Prayer, Laughter & Broccoli, A Breast Cancer Survival Guide for Husbands." Its revised second edition is now available. Peter was named a 2007 Breast Cancer Champion by Yoplait, Self Magazine, and the Susan G. Komen Foundation. He is a freelance writer and Relationship Manager with Heartland Payment Systems based in Connecticut. He has more than 35 years in the not-for-profit charitable sector. Peter and his wife Shirley speak nationwide on couples surviving and thriving the journey together. peterjflierl@gmail.com*

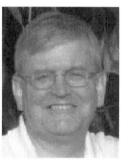

My bride of 34 years, Shirley Flierl, was diagnosed with breast cancer when she was 37 years old. Our daughter Alison was then 3 years of age. Shirley was facing a battle for her life. Alison and I were coping with what I believed and perhaps Alison sensed would likely be the loss of the most important person in both of our lives. Shirley was diagnosed with a Stage 3 aggressive breast tumor, one that was too large and too deep into her chest wall, to be completely removed. She had extensive lymph node involvement. Her clinical team—surgeon, oncologist, radiation therapist—did not believe she would be with us long term. Shirley experienced a year of aggressive treatment: six months of chemotherapy and hormone therapy, followed by six weeks of daily radiation therapy, then another six months of chemotherapy. We also ate broccoli literally every day, as it was the only vegetable Alison would eat.

When faced with this challenge, I did the unthinkable and asked for help. I had "special friends" who were always there for me. I had one magnificent friend, Louise Crisafi, who gave me some marvelous advice on how to be of help and how to support Shirley. From all around me, I drew strength, comfort, and understanding.

Then in 2010, Shirley was diagnosed again with breast cancer following her "routine" annual mammography. It was caught early, very small. It was not a recurrence and Shirley is recovering nicely. Life and loving go on as we celebrated 34 years of marriage in September. The common sense advise we used throughout our years together since the first diagnosis have provided us uncommon strength. I hope they help you and your partner.

When faced with this challenge, I did the unthinkable and asked for help. I had "special friends" who were always there for me. I had one magnificent friend, Louise Crisafi, who gave me some marvelous advice on how to be of help and how to support Shirley. From all around me, I drew strength, comfort, and understanding.

The common sense advise we used throughout our years together since the first diagnosis have provided us uncommon strength. I hope they help you and your partner.

### 1. Tell Her You Love Her

In a marriage or any intimate relationship, silence is not golden. The strong silent type need not apply for the position of husband, lover, best friend, confidante, caregiver and supporter of a woman with breast cancer. Your bride, your wife, needs and wants to hear from you. Actions may speak louder than words, and you may take all the right actions, but speaking words brings comfort, reassurance and knowledge of your inner feelings. She cannot read your mind. Being there for her is more than physical or economic security. Words have meaning. And the three most important words in the English language at this time, at this moment, when you together face her mortality, are: "I love you." The late Louise Crisafi, a saint here on Earth, always giving of herself for others in need, taught me this lesson on the Friday Shirley had her biopsy and was diagnosed, having opted for the then new two-step process. This meant we knew on Friday that she would have a mastectomy on Monday, a weekend together, scared, anxious, frightened. For Shirley, confronting death and permanent loss of part of her womanhood. For me, just at a loss and floundering, not knowing what to do or what to say. Louise was an American Cancer Society Reach to Recovery volunteer devoted to helping other women facing breast cancer diagnosis and treatment. She was a good friend. When I asked Louise what to do feeling as helpless and overwhelmed as I was, she said simply: "Tell her you love her." I was off to the races. I spent the weekend saying those magic, powerful words over and over, as frequently as possible, perhaps more than I had done in weeks, months or years previously. A year or so later in a television talk show featuring three women with breast cancer, including Louise, Shirley reminisced about how verbal I had become that fateful first weekend. Those words brought comfort and made a difference. Say, "I love you." It works.

### 2. Say "Yes"

We all know the classic joke about Moses and the tribes of Israel wandering for 40 years in the desert after their miraculous escape from bondage in Egypt. It took 40 long years to reach the land of milk and honey, the Promised Land. But why did it take so long? Moses was a man. He refused to ask for directions. Ten Commandments, maybe; asking for help, never. If you're married or even dated a man for any length of time, you've spent time in a car lost. You suggest, perhaps timidly and quietly, that it might be a good idea to stop and ask for directions. Louise Crisafi taught me to accept help when I asked her what to do knowing that Shirley and I were facing her cancer together, a cancer we had little hope of beating. Her advice was powerful, wise, and insightful. When someone, anyone, asks if they can do anything to help, just say: "Yes." Friends, neighbors, colleagues and others want to be there for you and for themselves. I know, I know. You're a man and never ask for help, not even simple directions. Understand that the people asking to help need your "Yes" as much as you. It gives them some sense of being able to do something positive about this insidious disease that seems beyond their control. Like you, they want to do something. Bottom line. Ask for help. Accept help. Say "yes" when it's offered. You'll be better for it and so will those seeking to be of service.

### 3. Laugh, Humor Heals

Norman Cousins taught the country this lesson about the healing power of humor many years ago and we are often reminded of this truth. We know that the act of laughing is healing. It makes us feel better and helps us get better. It is very easy to take ourselves in particular, our careers, and our work much too seriously. Close friends have experienced our occasional over-the-top, out of control laughing, true guffaws, and sometimes snorting. Does anything feel better? You cannot laugh while feeling sorry for yourself. Seeing the humor in any situation brings relief and release. Shirley set the stage for our approach to her treatment for breast cancer, which included large doses of humor from day one. As she was wheeled in for a mastectomy, laying on a gurney just outside the operating room, she looked up and said to her surgeon, Phil McWhorter: "Hey, Phil, you ought to charge me half price. I'm pretty small." She is the epitome of courage, strength, and fortitude. She was and is a winner.

A year later, Shirley suggested to the hospital's then President & CEO that she was being over charged for her mammogram, that she should get a 50% discount. After all, they only had to take a single x-ray image, not two. What's fair is fair. She left him speechless. It just makes sense to me. And there was her relationship with her oncologist, Dick Hollister, and his incredible office staff. Do you realize that over 95% of cancer treatment takes place in a physician's private office, not in a hospital? Dick and his staff always provided hope, comfort, and, best of all, large doses of laughter and humor. Dick had made the choice to become a doctor and treat patients with cancer at age 13. He was the perfect match for Shirley, who turned him bright red (fairly easy given his red-head's freckled complexion), when she whipped out her temporary breast prosthesis during his first visit to her hospital room. He was speechless. He knew he had a live one, despite the poor prognosis. Shirley was an interesting and challenging case for a new oncologist in his first few years of practice. Jokes were a staple in his office during the course of our year of treatment. Humor is healing to body, mind, and spirit.

## 4. Be faithful. Be monogamous.

We do not hear espoused or celebrated often enough the value and benefits of faithfulness, fidelity and monogamy. Nor do we hear of the sacred nature of marriage and its profound role in the social contract. A long term, monogamous relationship is exquisitely intimate. A good friend, a woman, said of my views on monogamy: "How quaint." As in charming, old fashioned, unusual or unfamiliar, even strange. And then I look at our role models, Shirley's parents, Art and Marge, were married for more than 69 years. That is the goal. We find in it our deepest nature, our essential and fundamental selves. We become acutely perceptive of each other in a relationship that is intense and keen. It is as delicate and beautiful as a snowflake, as hard and lustrous as a diamond. As a man, you will understand with certainty that your wife truly completes you in every way: physically, emotionally, and spiritually. You owe it to her and yourself to develop the depth of understanding brought on only by being faithful for life. God meant us as marriage partners to be one together for life. Swans do it, so can we.

## 5. I Love You, Not Your Breasts

Despite our nation's growing obesity, we are a breast and body image fixated society, from Betty Grable pinups in World War II, Marilyn Monroe and Jane Mansfield in the

1950's and 1960's to Salma Hayek and Pamela Anderson today. Men talk about being "leg men" or "breast men" with bravado and sophomoric stupidity, as if large breasts or great legs has anything at all to do with being a woman, or a lifetime companion, or a long-term intimate lover. Now, don't get me wrong. I still like to look at and admire beautiful women from the gorgeous 76-year-old former model in a smoking cessation class in 1982 to the stars and women around me.

However, it is my bride, my lover, and my lifetime partner who is my sexual and sensual interest today. Your bride, your lover, needs to know that you love who she is, not what type of body she has or the size of her breasts. Shirley is as beautiful and sexy today as she was on our first date. Our love making then and today was not and is not hampered by her having one breast instead of two. Rather, it enriches our intimacy. When we make love, she completes me, makes me whole and alive. Your bride needs reassurance in the face of an assault on her femininity and sense of womanhood. She needs to know by what you say and what you do that this set of circumstances is not the end of your sex life, but rather a new, sometimes frightening, and exciting sex life with heightened sensitivity and caring.

## 6. Go to Her Appointments

Go to the multitude of appointments with your wife, your partner, as much as you can, holding her hand literally and figuratively. In 1982, I had the luxury of relative independence in my 24/7 position as the CEO of an innovative and unique community health education and wellness center. I built my professional and community calendar around Shirley's treatment schedule. I went with Shirley to virtually every physician visit, every chemotherapy appointment. I felt a bit guilty about sitting in the waiting room, not going into the exam room with her for the actual treatments. Perhaps a bit of a wimp or squeamish, but I was with her in mind, body and spirit every step of the way. If it were possible, I would have taken it for her, traded places with her. It is not what you do when you accompany her to treatment, but rather the act itself that speaks volumes to her. It also gives you some sense of empowerment. You are more than a helpless spectator cursing the damned disease. You have joined the journey.There is also a practical side. Hearing a diagnosis of cancer overwhelms the senses. Doctors try to help you understand, but their daily jargon, the language of medicine, might as well be classical Greek or Latin. With two of you there, there are two sets of ears to hear what is said. There are two mouths to ask questions. This helps avoid the tendency to hear what you want to hear. Being with her each time will reassure her, help her overcome, and make you feel good about yourself. She'll love you for it.

## 7. Help With Your Child or Children

Shirley and I were blessed with our daughter, Alison, who was three years old when Shirley started treatment. Dick Hollister, her oncologist, gave us a choice following her surgery: the option of having more children or aggressive treatment that might save Shirley's life, a long shot at best, but a remote possibility. Our joint decision, our opting for her life, took a nanosecond. Raising Alison, being her mother, was Shirley's passionate mission. It was her reason for living and surviving. Your children need both of you. Depending on their age, they may or may not really understand what is happening, or share your anxiety and fears. They will know that something is amiss. They need you both. And she will need you to take over more and more as chemotherapy or radiation take their toll, making her tired and sick, taking away her energy and leaving her in need of rest. She is a warrior doing battle. To win ultimate victory, let her husband (what a marvelous word) be her strength and resources. She will do what she can. She will want to be involved. But you need to step in seamlessly when she needs down time. Can you give a greater gift?

## 8. Eat Your Broccoli

When you read any literature concerning breast cancer and nutrition, or other cancers and nutrition, you read about low fat diets and eating cruciferous vegetables. At the top of the list of vegetables most frequently mentioned is broccoli. At the time of Shirley's treatment, Alison loved broccoli and would eat no other vegetable, so we ate broccoli with dinner literally every night for the whole year of treatment. The first President Bush may not have eaten his broccoli, but it was good for us. It is not beyond the realm of possibility that daily consumption of broccoli enhanced treatment and contributed in some way to Shirley's survival. She suggested just that to her oncologist half jokingly and half seriously. He just shrugged his shoulders, acknowledging that we don't know. He is as surprised at her survival as we are joyful. Perhaps the daily broccoli regimen helped in some unknown way.

## 9. Sex and Recovery After Breast Cancer

I have spoken on this subject to women's groups and social workers. Most rewarding was being part of a panel in Stamford, Connecticut with a professional sex therapist speaking ahead of me. I listened attentively and was pleased to find that Shirley and I had figured out on our own what she described in theory. She was a theoretician explaining the principles underlying sexuality and the impact of breast surgery and cancer treatment. Shirley and I had lived it and muddled through on our own just fine, thank you. This is another place where a man needs to let his partner lead. She will let you know what works now and what doesn't, what she's ready for, and what she's not. I suppose I mourned the loss of her breast as she did, as well as the change in some aspects of lovemaking that resulted. The important thing to learn is that life goes on and sex goes on. In the first weeks, months and even years, your sex life may take on an added dimension that is simultaneously painful and exquisite. Imagine how it feels to make love to someone you feel you might lose. You don't want to hurt her. Remember, she is not fragile. You can give her bear hugs both during and outside your lovemaking.

One of the best things for us was a marvelous gynecologist who discussed sexual issues with Shirley and had a number of practical suggestions. Most important was "the stuff used by prostitutes in Stamford" to be used by us to make intercourse more comfortable for her. A blessing. Yes, there is both life and sex during and after treatment for breast cancer. Your partner, your bride, knows how she can best deal with her breast cancer. In Shirley's case, she opted for minimal information from day one. She chose to rely on Dick Hollister and Joe Murphy to let her know how she was doing in the simplest of ways. Good or bad blood count, for example, not the numbers, not analysis. There is no "right" way or "wrong" way. It is her way, her journey, her path. Some patients with cancer try to become oncologists in a heartbeat, reading, reading, and reading more medical literature. Seeking out more and more information, perhaps seeking second, third and fourth opinions. Others may rely on their physician, a man or woman dedicated to healing and life, to be their coach and guide them through the process. Whatever path you choose is the right path for you. Shirley was the Joe Friday of cancer patients, asking for the facts, nothing but the facts. And keep it short and simple. Shirley did not feel a need to hear or be given all the numbers from her ongoing testing, retesting and testing again. She chose to rely on her physicians, particularly Dick Hollister and Phil McWhorter and their staff, to keep her current with the simplest of terms. Was a blood count good or bad, for example? She did not need or want to hear the numbers. She did not want to analyze her situation. Other women may opt to become overnight medical students or aspiring physicians, trying to learn in an instant what a physician has studied and absorbed over eight years or more. For Shirley and for me, despite my being a clinical social worker and a "health care professional," simple was best. A sound physician-patient relationship is built on mutual respect and trust. It enhances your healing.

## 10. Anger

Let your anger out. Shirley was very little on the "why me" or "poor me" approach to her disease and her treatment. She was angry about the thought of not seeing Alison grow up. What did matter were survival, good health, and living into our dotage. Or, at least until Alison grew up, went through college, and perhaps started a family along with pursuing her dream of writing and directing films. In other words, Shirley's passion, her overriding concern, was to be a mother to her daughter, her only child. The one and only thought that brought her to venting her anger was the possibility of not seeing Alison grow up. Shirley vented her rage in our kitchen sink. She threw old glasses into the sink, smashing them one by one, and having a good cry. Very satisfying. Quite cathartic. My preference was pounding the steering wheel while driving the car and sobbing. It's OK. The point is that anger is OK, as long as it doesn't cripple you. Living life fully and passionately relieves the anger.

## Final Thought—Pay It Forward

Shirley was led through her treatment and recovery by a friend, the late Louise Crisafi, an American Cancer Society Reach to Recovery volunteer. Louise and I worked closely together, she as a volunteer serving on my board of directors and me as staff, so it was natural that both Shirley and I turned to her for support, direction, comfort and understanding. Most important, we needed her faith, her profound rock solid belief in a caring, compassionate Christian God. Like most Reach to Recovery volunteers, Louise gave Shirley hope, belief that she could beat her cancer. She helped Shirley through the process of choosing between having a one-step or a two-step biopsy and surgery. She let me know what I could do to be of help. She visited. She called. She was a presence in our lives, particularly Shirley's. Shirley wondered what she could do to repay her and Louise's response was to pass it on to another woman in need, to pay it forward as demonstrated so beautifully in the recent movie by that name. Shirley chose 28 years ago, in an era when breast cancer was just beginning to come out of the closet, to be public and open about her disease and her treatments. That was a fateful decision that over the years has saved others lives, women who knew her or knew of her, who finally decided to have their mammograms and checkups. Her openness and willingness to serve others brought and continues to bring countless phone calls from women who need and want to talk it through. When Louise had a recurrence that ultimately took her life, we confided in each other. She was one of the first civilians with whom I shared my personal battle with alcoholism, also a terminal disease, and my day-to-day recovery, now having lasted an amazing 32 years. It was a shared bond felt by both of us. I kept my life and keep my life by giving it away.

# 20.
# The Unlikely Muse Called Cancer

## BY JACKIE FOX

*Jackie Fox is a writer and breast cancer thriver who lives in Nebraska with her
husband Bruce. She blogs about breast cancer, gratitude, humor and life at
http://secondbasedispatch.com and is author of the book "From Zero to Mastectomy:
What I Learned and You Need to Know About Stage 0 Breast Cancer".*

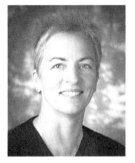

**B**efore I was diagnosed with breast cancer, the last word I would have associated with it is "muse." Yet that's exactly what cancer became for me. Reconnecting with friends and family is a more obvious example of the benefits cancer can bring, but old loves like art and literature may reappear in your life as well. In my case, I started writing poetry again after a nearly 20-year absence and I don't know how to attribute it to anything but cancer.

I've always loved reading and writing poetry. I wrote about my paternal grandmother Rose in fifth grade, taking a bit of creative license and turning her into a fairy. I wrote typically mushy poetry in high school and got bètter when I took poetry writing in college. I took classes from two different professors, one of whom edits a highly regarded Midwestern poetry journal. She told me I needed to push myself and take graduate classes, which I did not, but I'm thinking about it now. That's the wonderful thing about learning and writing—there's no time limit.

Back then, I got a handful of things published in an anthology about grandmothers (Rose again—this time, it didn't rhyme) in poetry journals that no longer exist, and in Rolling Stone magazine—back in the day, they used to include poetry as well as music reviews. They even paid me $10 per poem! (Even today, you're most likely to be paid in copies.)

I don't mean to imply that getting published is the be all and end all. It's certainly nice, but what really matters is the joy of creating. Whether it's hearing a story that makes your inner tuning fork go off so you grab a pen in the middle of a cocktail party or business meeting, or feeling the poem flow through you like automatic writing, it's a rush.

I had all that. And then it left me. I don't know why, but I didn't think about attempting to write poetry and barely thought about reading it for nearly 20 years. I missed it, but it didn't occur to me to do anything to try to get it back. I really believed that part of my life was over.

Then something happened. I don't know why it started again any more than I know why it stopped, but I can only believe the muse came back disguised as cancer.

First, poems started speaking to me again. I'll never forget the day I realized I didn't want to gamble with my life. It was June 11, 2008. When my husband and I left my oncologist's office after he recommended a mastectomy, I was reeling. To top it off, there were tornados all around the Omaha area that night. We spent a good two hours in our designated tornado room when we usually spend 40 minutes at most. The next day, I came across a poem in The New Yorker by Franz Wright called "*The Realm of the Senses.*" The first stanza took my breath away:

"What a day. I had some trouble
following the plot line; however,
the special effects were incredible."

He couldn't have spoken any more directly to me if he had sent me a text message. I saved the poem.

Next, poems started speaking through me again. We went to Cabo san Lucas in November for our first real vacation in more than a year. I had three surgeries under my belt and was a couple of weeks away from my second stage reconstruction and augmentation.

While we were in Cabo, something took place that put me squarely in mind of the G.K. Chesterton quote, "Coincidences are spiritual puns." We went to an Italian restaurant on the harbor that happened to have a wonderful jazz singer, Daline Jones, performing for her new CD launch party. Just listening to her was wonderful and all was right with the world like it always is when you hear great music.

Then something amazing happened. She started reciting a poem, "Truth," which I hadn't thought of for more than 30 years. Turns out her dad wrote it. It was one of my high-school favorites and before I knew it, I was reciting along with her. I started clapping like you do for a great jazz solo but since this was a poem I was the only one clapping. Our table was pretty close to the stage, and she turned to me and bowed. I bowed back. I was beyond blown away.

I had written my first poem in all those years a couple of weeks before the trip (which I recently found out is going to be published in an anthology of Nebraska women poets), and the weekend we got back, I wrote four new poems and reworked an old one. I felt like gift upon gift was piling up.

I've written more than three dozen poems (or at least drafts) since then. Three of them were inspired by my excellent breast cancer adventure, but most were not. I've sent some of them to different venues that publish poetry. Six of them have been accepted for publication and many more have been rejected. Whether I find homes for more of them or not, I'm having a great time.

My best guess at why the muse came back is that I realized there's no time to waste. Cancer is definitely a wake-up call, even if it's caught early like mine was. Perhaps a bigger but related reason is that I let go of something. A friend told me as much; she said she could see it in my face.

To be honest, I let go of quite a few things. I let go of my physical modesty when I had to present the girls for inspection to at least one of my four doctors on a weekly basis. I let go of the usual niggling worries that seemed big until the overwhelming presence called cancer showed up and crowded them out. I let go of my mistaken belief that I was in control. And I let go of fear. Maybe I needed to let go of all those things to make room for the muse.

## 21.

# From Surviving to Thriving: How I Quit Thinking of Cancer as My Diagnosis

### BY AMELIA FRAHM

*Amelia Frahm helped pioneer resources for children affected by cancer. She's the owner of Nutcracker Publishing Company, author of the award winning "Tickles Tabitha's Cancer-tankerous Mommy", and creator of the Crack Open a Book! cancer education curriculum for elementary school children. Her next book, "How a Nuclear Power Plant Really Works" is scheduled to be completed in 2011. For info: www.nutcrackerpublishing.com. Amelia@nutcrackerpublishing.com / 919-924-2058*

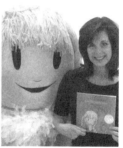

Sitting on the sofa in my great room, I watched as my children raced to see who would reach me first. My 4-year old daughter, Tabitha, shoved her brother, Jordan, 2, out of the way and jumped feet first onto my lap. She was wearing a tutu and cowboy boots. Instinctively, I put up a hand to protect myself, and I felt a lump the size of an acorn in my breast. With a touch of my fingertips, my promising future had turned into a worried question mark. I was 34 years old and one pivotal moment had changed my life forever.

Breast cancer ended life as I knew it, the one in which I wrote excellent when asked to fill out health forms and believed bad things happened to other people. But I know now if breast cancer is the worst thing that ever happens to me, I'll be a lucky woman.

Today, I'm considered a pioneer in the field of talking to children about cancer. I'm the author of *Tickles Tabitha's Cancer-tankerous Mommy,* creator of the Crack Open a Book! cancer education curriculum for elementary school children, and owner of Nutcracker Publishing Company. I'll soon publish my second book. A children's book on nuclear power plants, based on experience obtained from my very first professional job which was doing public relations at a nuclear plant.

My journey has been long and up-hill, but the challenges, failures, heartbreak, and what at first glance appeared to be rotten luck, are what taught me to thrive. It took not only my own cancer, but the cancer diagnosis of a close friend before I quit fantasizing about what I wished would happen in my life and decided to make it happen. Along the way, I quit thinking of cancer as my diagnosis and began to regard it as my career.

As a breast cancer survivor, I learned that one moment can change your life forever, and as a breast cancer thriver, I learned to make the most of every moment left.

Intuitively I had known my lump was not "nothing to worry about," as the surgeon my primary doctor sent me to had suggested. He pointed out that I was healthy, not over-weight, had no family history of breast cancer, and my hair didn't require dye yet. After the biopsy he said he had seen nothing suspicious.

I lived then in Tennessee, and most of my friends and all of our family members lived in other states. I had just hung up the phone, after calling every single one of them to say I was okay, when my surgeon phoned to say he was sorry, but he'd been wrong. The pathologist's report said I had cancer. With that phone call I learned to appreciate words like mundane, and routine. I wanted my life to go back to being ordinary.

It was 1994, and my family and I could count the number of cancer survivors we knew on one hand. I felt as if I had been told I would not get to watch my children grow up, and I was devastated.

I had been convalescing on my bed while my children played nearby, and they witnessed their mommy fall apart. I can still picture the concern on their small faces. Jordan was too young to understand, but Tabitha was perceptive even then and wise beyond her years. She replenished cool, damp cloths for me and asked, if I had run out of tears yet.

I decided to be grateful it was me with cancer, and not one of my babies, so I dried my tears and determined I wouldn't be remembered as a hysterical wimp. Of course, I still cried... but I cried in my shower where no one could see me.

When a loved one dies, you grieve for one important person you have loved, but when you are the one dying, you realize you must say goodbye to every person you care about.

It didn't matter how many loved ones kept me company, I still felt alone; they couldn't die with me. It was then I understood the importance of believing in a higher power. I quit viewing my childhood Sunday school as a punishment and saw it for the gift it had been. You're never alone if you have faith in a higher power.

A well-endowed friend confided how sorry she was and how agonizing it must have been for me to decide to have a mastectomy. I laughed, because opting for a mastectomy was one of the easiest decisions I have ever made. All I had to do was think about the two small children I wanted to see grow up.

It's almost too bad for my family that I couldn't live the rest of my life like I did the weeks following my breast cancer diagnosis. I was kind, patient, and less demanding than I had ever been. Facing your own mortality really magnifies the best in a person. Or the worst! It wasn't long before my halo disappeared, and the Cancer-tankerous Mommy pictured in my children's book introduced herself. I have concluded since that survivors do not thrive by making life comfortable for the people around them.

All of us will encounter circumstances we must survive. They may be earth-shattering events such as cancer, unemployment, divorce, or the death of a child, or simply instances that force us to confront our own personal fears. I've had to confront my fear of needles and public speaking.

Thrivers don't use what we're surviving as an excuse. We use it as our motivation and inspiration to do something about our predicament. Even if at first, all it means is we have the courage to get out of bed each morning.

Breast cancer brought predicaments I never imagined. I was diagnosed when the word cancer was whispered above the heads of children, but I decided not to tiptoe around my diagnosis. Whispering upset my children and implied that my cancer was something to be embarrassed about. I decided not to allow whispering, or fibbing. I answered my children's questions honestly. I couldn't promise not to die, but I promised I would love them forever.

Breast cancer also brought issues that left me feeling guilty and ashamed. Like the way I behaved around my children. My prognosis was good, but my attitude did not reflect my gratitude. I was moody, short tempered and depressed.

I took out my frustrations on the people closest to me. In my opinion, the worst thing in the world is not surviving cancer; it is surviving the family member surviving it.

If my husband was optimistic, I was mad. Didn't he realize I could die? If he wasn't optimistic, I was still mad. Didn't he have faith I was going to live? I was on an emotional roller coaster and my children were seated behind me. I am grateful that when you've been diagnosed with cancer people, especially children tend to forgive you no matter how crazy you behave.

In hindsight, I realized that when I was finally able to write, and talk about my disease without apology, I began to thrive. I didn't grow my backbone overnight. It took years.

When I was diagnosed, the Internet was in its infancy. I couldn't Google "breast cancer," but I could visit the library. I had checked out children's books on potty training and sibling rivalry, so I was surprised to find no books to help explain my cancer craziness to my children.

Still crazy, but undaunted, I went home and wrote my own story. It didn't just help my children, it helped me. I noticed that celebrity survivors had made breast cancer advocacy popular on the evening news, and I figured the time had come for a children's book about it. I sent my manuscript to large, mainstream publishers who responded with rejection letters that also said my "wonderful, poignant, heart-warming story, sadly, needed to be told." Just not by them!

I assumed they were being nice because I was sick. I know now how naïve that sounds. Large publishing houses do not show mercy.

Mine was a niche topic, and as one editor advised, there were just not enough young moms with cancer to justify the expense of publishing and marketing such a book. The editor was wrong, but I didn't know enough to disagree.

I thought rejection was the last thing I needed, so I put my manuscript away and channeled my energy into surviving. It would take my friend Laura's cancer diagnosis five years later, before I found the courage to take that manuscript out of the closet.

Laura Bouldin Karlman was my best friend. We'd met in our early 20's before husbands, children, and careers took our lives in different directions. A registered nurse, Laura had been there for me during my cancer and now she had leukemia. I had moved to Minnesota and she was in Texas, but we spent hours on the phone, reminiscing, and confiding in each other. Laura had two children, and I learned with relief that I was not the only sick mommy who sometimes acted mean, moody in front of her kids.

Laura and I also discovered it was the very things that had left us paralyzed by fear and crimson with embarrassment, like the fools we had been during our dating years, that on death's door we did not regret one bit, but laughed about most.

I vowed I would not die regretting I had not tried to accomplish one of my secret ambitions because I feared failure, or ridicule, or someone told me I couldn't do it, no matter how logical the reason.

I'm often asked about my "a-ha: moment, when I knew I would change how I lived my life.

That moment came at MD Anderson Cancer Center in Houston, where I had gone to say a final good bye to Laura.

When I found out Laura had cancer I also discovered there was still not a children's book about cancer for young women and/or families coping with the issues surrounding it. So I took another look at my manuscript.

Laura had encouraged me to publish my book, and knew mainstream publishers had rejected it. What she did not know was that just before my trip to Texas I had borrowed several thousand dollars and established an independent publishing company to publish the book myself. Something I knew nothing about. Nor did she know what I had decided to call my company. By the time I arrived in Texas she was too sick to hear about my plans.

Laura, her mother, sisters and I had a slumber party in her hospital room where we talked, cried and laughed. To this day I feel privileged to have been included.

Even sick, Laura could be stubborn. She did something that aggravated her youngest sister, who called Laura a "nut," which was a tame insult for her. But perhaps because Laura was dying, she appeared to rethink even that and added the word "cracker," saying "Laura, you're just a nutcracker."

This was my sign. I knew then and there I would do what I was meant to do—publish my book. The name I had given my company was Nutcracker Publishing. A fitting name as I knew my friends and family would think I was nuts.

Laura died October 27, 2000, at 39 years old. Less than two years after her cancer diagnosis. My company is dedicated to her memory.

One year later, Nutcracker Publishing released *Tickles Tabitha's Cancer-tankerous Mommy*.

Despite overwhelming odds, a niche topic, and an author with zero consumer recognition within its first year, *Tickles Tabitha's Cancer-Tankerous Mommy* earned the acclaim of health care organizations and advocates across the country, including the National Oncology Nursing Society, Rosie O'Donnell, and the Susan G. Komen Foundation.

There were still tremendous ups and downs and surviving cancer had been good preparation for them. An upset stomach and nausea were nothing new to me, so once again I took my medicine. This time instead of a pill, it came in the form of rejection, from people who did not appreciate my book idea.

Sometimes the ups and down occurred on the same day , such as when my book went to print and then my mother called to say she had been diagnosed with breast cancer. Following that came 9/11, the threat of anthrax, and the Iraq War, all of which affected my one-woman company.

I had won what, for any author, much less an unknown, first-time, non-celebrity one, was the publisher's lottery when I was invited to appear on Rosie O' Donnell's TV show to announce my book's release and help celebrate October's Breast Cancer Awareness Month.

Then terrorists struck the Twin Towers in New York City where the show aired. Despite that, its producers decided the show would go on. Many Americans were afraid to fly, especially to New York City, so word about my plans was big news near my Minnesota home and in many of the small Southern towns I had resided previously. Quite a few newspaper articles had been written about me.

I'll always remember the phone call I received from my father, who begged me not to fly to New York. His prayers were answered, because the day before my departure anthrax was found at the studio where the show aired and my appearance was canceled. The hometown hero had been shoved off her author's pedestal by a bacteria. It was very disappointing, but one thing I had learned from my cancer diagnosis was how to get through a crisis.

And I did get through it. Although I didn't appear on Rosie O'Donnell's show, my book did, and she recommended it on the air. I might not have known much about publishing, but I had a degree in public relations. My first professional job had been to explain the virtues of nuclear power, right after the Three Mile Island incident and during the Chernobyl accident. I put that experience to work and wrote a press release about my book surviving anthrax.

The story was picked up by the Associated Press, and calls trickled in from across the country. As one radio host said over the air, laughing: "We heard you weren't going to be going to New York City, and thought maybe you'd be free to do our show."

What would probably have been a forgotten author appearance became a story of national interest. Soon, I became a nationally recognized author/expert, not just on talking to children about cancer, but on small press publishing, marketing, and how to turn a public relations lemon into lemonade. Later that year, I was honored to be invited to join the National Cancer Survivor's Day Speakers Bureau, among celebrity cancer survivors.

The news was ironic because before my cancer, one of my biggest personal fears was public speaking. As I now tell my audiences, "when I was in college I was so shy I took a failing grade rather than get up in front of the class and introduce myself.  Pretty much everything I've claimed was a waste of time because I was afraid to do it, I've now done, been or married."

Not long ago, I stared out at the bewildered faces of an elementary school class during another of my author visits. I tried to explain to the reality TV generation that when I first published *Tickles Tabitha's Cancer-tankerous Mommy*, talking about cancer to my own children had raised eyebrows, and taking the book to a class like theirs was unimaginable.

My ideas have not always been greeted enthusiastically, and even today my cancer education program for children is often met with resistance. I know I'm not a wacko; I'm just a step ahead of popular perception.

Now I'm focused on my children's book about nuclear power plants, another niche topic, and that familiar feeling in the pit of my stomach has returned. I never would have had the audacity to write and publish this book had I not suffered from cancer.

Life is full of self-doubt, fear of failure and nervous queasiness, but I am no longer paralyzed by these feelings. They are the emotions of a survivor, and once I conquer them again, I will look back with the sweet satisfaction of a thriver.

A few months ago, I pulled a chest muscle while water-skiing and feared at first that I had ruptured one of the implants from my reconstructive surgery.

It turned out my implant was fine, but my daughter smiled as she told me, "Those implants are old." I realized that my doctors had never discussed replacing the implants because they didn't think I would live long enough to make it necessary.

One moment can change a life forever. This one reminded me I am still thriving.

# 22.
# Survivor vs. Thriver: What's the Difference?

## BY KERRI GEARY

*Kerri James Geary – Educator, Speaker, Journey Practitioner, and Spiritual Mentor—
is no stranger to health care. She experienced primary breast cancer twice and endured a
plethora of medical procedures including several major surgeries, a ridiculous assortment
of scans and x-rays, and way too many blood draws to count! Her loved ones affectionately
call her The Bionic Woman. "We can rebuild her, we have the technology!" As a result of her
experiences, Kerri is enthusiastically devoted to serving others as a healing guide during
any or all stages of the healing process. By combining real world experience in both allopathic
(Western) and complementary medicine with her training in holistic stress management,
mind/body preparation for medical procedures, emotional processing, and spiritual
exploration, she is able to meet specific individual needs. She lives in Fort Collins,
Colorado with her husband, Mike, and son, Evan. Kerri welcomes questions and
can be reached by phone by e-mail, kerri@compassionateembrace.com.*

When two people face a similar traumatic experience, why is it that one person is able to thrive while the other descends into feelings of despair, self-pity, or bitterness? As a breast cancer survivor (twice!), I've discovered that healing from trauma requires more than merely regaining physical wellness. The transformation from surviving into thriving occurs when we engage with life, connect with others, and open ourselves to the enormous possibilities available for healing. This metamorphosis can occur quickly or proceed slowly over a long period of time. And, just like everything else in life, the 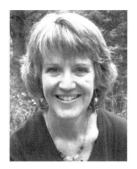 degree to which people experience and overcome trauma happens on a continuum from barely surviving to genuinely thriving.

My understanding of the various dimensions of thriving after trauma flows from an ongoing exploration of both my father's health challenges as well as my own. Only after experiencing trauma myself did I recognize that what my father endured included elements of transcendence as well as suffering. I realize now that watching him cope with the pain, anxiety, and outright terror that often accompany a life-threatening diagnosis helped prepare me to face the health issues that eventually confronted me. Hopefully, the insights I have gained about how we thrived after our traumas will help you discover your own path to thriving.

I used to believe that a person could only thrive if they had good physical health, yet this belief unraveled as I witnessed my father's soul expand, even as his body began to disintegrate. Having an uncooperative body that prohibited robust physical activity was apparently not a prerequisite for my dad's thriving. Handsome, outgoing, athletic, and enterprising, Dad appeared to "have it all" and enjoyed both his work and home life. A larger-than-life sort of guy, he tended to be the main attraction in most situations and seemed to be both lucky and blessed, at least until the age of 43, when doctors discovered a cancerous tumor in his sinus cavity. His malignancy diagnosis forever altered both his life and mine.

With the seriousness of the cancer, the doctors speculated that my Dad might survive only a few years. Fortunately for our family, the doctors' prognosis simply did not fit with my dad's plans. He lived nineteen more years, despite the horrendous effects of massive radiation to his head, resulting in the loss of his eyesight, hearing in one ear, most of his teeth, and much of his dignity. Even though his strong body deteriorated over time, my father's stubborn will, sense of humor, and desire to provide for his family kept him going.

Before the cancer treatment, my father often judged people by their appearance and didn't notice when or if he hurt someone's feelings with his "harmless" teasing. He could be chauvinistic, bossy, and quick-tempered, with little patience and quite a bit of arrogance. After the cancer treatment, none of these characteristics served him well, and so these traits gradually fell away, replaced by qualities that opened his heart and matured his soul. These new attributes arose out of a combination of necessity, deep contemplation, and inherited values such as hard work, perseverance, and the importance of community service.

The first change that I noticed was that, without sight, Dad no longer judged people by their looks. Consequently, his connections with others became more positive, more authentic. When asked about his health, my father always shifted the focus of the conversation back to the other person, resulting in that person feeling cared about and acknowledged. Although he often had pain or discomfort, Dad never wanted to talk about himself and didn't dwell on his own problems. Little did I realize that his defiant response to his cancer diagnosis would provide me with tremendous lessons for coping with my own health issues!

As my father wiled away umpteen hours with only his mind for company, he immersed himself in deep contemplation about life, other people, and the difficulties going on in the world. He could have chosen to shut down, sitting in silence or sleeping all the time, but instead he preoccupied himself with creative problem solving and thought-provoking inquiries, offering expertise and ideas to a variety of individuals and organizations. My dad also continued to attend business and social functions all the way up to his last few months alive, remaining engaged with life even as his body was preparing to leave it. Despite being burdened with degenerating health, my Dad lived a life that remains a true testament to thriving.

Dad's numerous interfaces with the medical world also nurtured other supportive qualities. As he encountered people dealing with trauma in countless doctor's offices and hospitals, his compassion progressively grew. Forced to wait for appointments, rides, test results, and just about everything else including his meals, Dad learned to be a "patient" patient. In the face of death and in the midst of pain and suffering, my father also acquired the requisite courage needed to sustain him through a variety of frightening medical procedures and experiences. I believe this courage stemmed from an inner knowing that he was more than just a body, as well as a deep desire to thrive in spite of all his difficulties.

Having almost died four times during post-cancer treatment, my father felt thankful every single day for the sublime pleasure of simply waking up alive. This gratitude helped him stay centered in the present moment, where life really happens and flourishes. He let go of the past and didn't worry about the future, remaining open to all the possibilities of the "now." Dad trusted and knew that God was present, and his humility in dealing with the profound changes in his life circumstances touched and inspired all of us who knew and loved him. Like Christopher Reeve, Michael J. Fox, and Roger Ebert, my father exemplified the essence of thriving in the face of severe physical limitations. Sadly, Dad passed away in 1994, but the inner resources that he cultivated throughout his nearly 20 years of emotional and physical suffering provided me with solid ground to stand on as I confronted my own health challenges. In fact, the lessons he taught me continue to resonate through virtually every aspect of my life to this very day.

As I matured, my father's circumstances with cancer impacted me immensely, in both positive and negative ways. In the aftermath of my father's diagnosis, during that crazy, volatile time of changing from a girl into a young woman, I developed numerous unhealthy habits and ways of coping that I carried forth well into my adult life. The news of my father's cancer and the wrenching changes that it brought about stirred up many unfamiliar emotions that I didn't know how to express, and certainly didn't want to feel anyway.

These emotions had nothing to do with what I considered "good" feelings. Therefore, I tried not to have them, forcing the feelings back into my body, daydreaming, and using drugs and alcohol. I had no idea that this unhealthy coping mechanism of "numbing out" was the beginning of a lifelong pattern of emotional suppression. Disintegrating into different parts, completely unaware of losing my sense of wholeness, I meandered mindlessly through my teen years while struggling with both depression and with what I perceived as the superficialities of high school in America.

In an attempt to escape the pain of my home life, I chose to attend a university over a thousand miles away, literally running away from my problems. During my time at college, I began to feel alive and happy again, excelling in academics and slowly allowing my heart to open a little more each year. After college graduation, I joined the Peace Corps and spent two years in Sierra Leone, West Africa, living in a small village, enjoying a totally different culture, and feeling satisfied about making friends and helping less fortunate people. What I didn't realize at the time is that I became a volunteer to avoid my emotional pain, having placed it on an imaginary shelf while living as far away from home as I could possibly get.

Once my two-year commitment to the Peace Corps ended, I returned to the U.S. and began working as an elementary school teacher. Marriage soon followed, and within a few years, I settled into what I thought was a contented existence of work, home life, and the occasional travel adventure. Despite this semblance of "normalcy," the truth is that I was still ignoring the emotional baggage of my childhood, dragging it along with me like a ball and chain while neglecting my emotional needs as an adult. It seems the life of denial I was leading had put both my physical and emotional health in a precarious situation.

When doctors discovered cancer in my right breast at age 32, I remember thinking about my father's ability to thrive in a battered body, which definitely helped me cope with the devastating news. Having only been exposed to traditional western medicine and feeling terrified by the ramifications of a cancer diagnosis, I simply couldn't conceive of disobeying the recommendations of my doctors, nor did I consider that other, perhaps less destructive healing possibilities existed. So, I accepted what I thought was my fate and underwent a complete mastectomy and TRAM flap reconstruction, which was considered the "gold standard" of surgery at that time.

To put it bluntly, the TRAM flap reconstruction I endured was extremely traumatic. Reconstruction is actually a bit of a misnomer; my entire being felt utterly violated! My recovery from this painful, invasive surgery took many months and even now, more than fourteen years later, my body is still dealing with the adverse effects of having my body parts rearranged.

Despite the trauma I had endured, my trusty habit of smothering my emotions took over and I once again managed to numb myself to the most intense feelings churning deep within. Over the ensuing years, I outwardly projected an optimistic veneer and went through my life as if nothing had ever happened, as if the cancer treatment were just a cold that I needed to get over. When I reached the widely recognized 5-year cancer benchmark, my oncologist declared me cured (yep, he actually used the "cure" word!). On top of that fabulous news, within a few months I discovered that I was pregnant with my first child at the ripe old age of 38. Life finally seemed to be getting back to normal, or at the very least, somewhat less traumatic!

Unfortunately, at a routine oncology check up three years later, and only several days after deciding to try for another child at age 41 (definitely pushing the envelope for conceiving, but what did I care, I simply adored being a Mom!), I received a diagnosis of a new primary breast cancer in my opposite breast. This time the news absolutely shattered my world. Not only was the cancer more invasive than the first one, but more importantly, I was a Mommy! I was a Mommy!!!! I felt like an enormous tornado had just swept me up and tossed me asunder. I couldn't breathe or sleep or even think clearly. I lost control of all hope and plummeted into an abyss of abject fear and unmitigated confusion.

After my first cancer experience, I had created a "healing toolbox" containing an assortment of tools to help me cope with my diagnosis, including supportive books, guided imagery CDs, and calming breath practices. This time around, however, I couldn't even manage to locate the toolbox, much less open it! Overwhelming feelings of despair soon paralyzed me. As the mother of a small child, this second cancer diagnosis only magnified my fear of the unknown. What would happen to my son if I didn't survive this time? How could I leave my husband to deal with raising a three year-old child alone?

Other strong emotions accompanied this intense fear. I experienced grief at the thought of putting my body through more violations, as well as a profound sense of betrayal: it all seemed so unfair! Perhaps most ominously, and completely unbeknownst to me, an all-consuming rage began boiling deep in the interior of my soul. Rage at cancer in general, rage at cancer in me, and rage at life itself! With all my strength, I tried to control these emotions by keeping them completely repressed, yet the energy required for this effort created an unbelievable level of anxiety and fatigue.

My oncologist put me on an anti-depressant, which dissipated the fear and partially abated the power of the rage. My school district gave me a one year leave-of-absence as I managed to make it through two more surgeries and chemotherapy, all while mothering a three year-old. The handful of resources that I had witnessed my father use to cope with his illness—like patience, optimism, and staying connected to others—served me well too, but nothing I had discovered so far helped me deal with the feelings boiling inside me.

The rage finally got my attention as the date of an impending surgery neared. I acquired a severe case of hives ALL OVER my body. I tried everything to alleviate the hives, but nothing worked until I experienced *The Journey*, a guided introspection process developed by Brandon Bays to promote cellular healing. Just one process quelled the screaming hives, and after two more sessions, my hives disappeared FOREVER! More significantly than that—and believe me, the significance of being hive-free cannot be understated—I had finally discovered a way to get in touch with my emotions and my soul. Brandon's guided introspection process empowered me with the emotional tools I needed to unify my heart, mind, body, and spirit.

In one of my most powerful processes, I realized that I had unwittingly given cancer its own consciousness, a sinister personality with malevolent intentions. This realization enabled me to disengage from the drama I had created around cancer. After that process, the question of "why?" began slipping from my vocabulary, replaced with the invitation, "Tell me more, body! What would you like me to learn? What are these cancer cells trying to communicate?"

As I began listening to my body and gradually developed an understanding of cellular healing, holistic medicine, and quantum physics, the most powerful lesson I learned is that by becoming numb to my emotions, I had essentially cut myself off from the infinite wisdom of my soul. My body used cancer to send me the urgent message that my whole being was out of balance in a multitude of ways. I also discovered that our bodies act as barometers for our emotions. Therefore, when we allow ourselves to experience our emotions fully, we are able to connect with our inner wisdom, receiving information critical to our complete health and well-being.

The guided introspection processes I learned through *The Journey* enabled me to uncover the hidden emotional blocks that my ego had created for my own safety, but that no longer served my highest potential. By eliminating these blocks, which had prevented me from fully healing and being consciously aware and alive, I was able to experience the direct connection between listening to my body and the process of cellular healing, which allowed me to extricate a lifetime of cancer consciousness from my entire being.

Working with my invaluable family practitioner, Dr. Jackie Fields, I also learned how to prevent the growth of cancer cells by balancing my "cellular terrain." Dr. Fields writes:

*Cancer is the abnormal growth of cells that rapidly replicate in the body when the body's house cleaning mechanisms do not function correctly, which allows the cells to develop a life and growth of their own. The development of abnormal cells actually occurs many times throughout our life. When the body's terrain is healthy, our body's house cleaning mechanisms take care of these abnormal cells so tumors do not develop. All types of cancer can be affected and even possibly prevented if we work hard to keep our cellular terrain and our beliefs healthy.*

Through adding or eliminating certain foods and supplements in my diet, I have strengthened my immune system, alkalized my pH levels, detoxified heavy metals from my organs, increased my blood viscosity, balanced my estrogen pathways, and supplied my cells with the appropriate nutrients for them to work properly. Now that I know which ingredients in both food and body products prevent cells from working properly, I have also become an avid label reader, which has led to wiser choices at the grocery store. Improving the functioning of all of these components has greatly improved my overall health and quality of life.

Bearing witness to my father's cancer journey encouraged me to explore the vast array of healing options currently available, options that range from prayer and meditation to guided imagery, from creative expression and holistic stress management techniques to emotional processing for cellular healing and complementary medicine. Unfortunately, my father did not have access to the incredible variety of healing opportunities open to me. Instead, he had to learn how to thrive the hard way, through trial-and-error and the rigors of "on-the-job" training, but I'm ever so proud of him for thriving in spite of all the obstacles he faced.

By embracing and welcoming all of my emotions and the entirety of my life circumstances, including cancer, my focus has shifted from the mundane details of everyday survival to the infinite beauty of this human experience. My purpose now is to share what I have learned with others who are facing traumatic experiences, in the sincere hope that they too can transform from merely surviving to genuinely thriving. As we open our hearts to love and actively connect with life itself by living in the present moment, we thrive and grow, prospering in the interior of our being while feeling extraordinarily healthy and vibrant. When you embrace the truth of who you are and learn to love that truth, everything else will flow, improving your chances to survive and thrive. Blessings for your healing journey!

# 23.

# Nancy Gratz Believes in Hope

## BY BEVERLY VOTE

*Nancy Gratz enjoys community work and meeting new people. She serves on the boards of the Cole County American Cancer Society and the Community Breast Care Project Board. She is an active member of the Chamber of Commerce. She is Past President of United Way, the Boys and Girls Club and Jefferson City Breakfast Rotary. She was honored to receive the Zonta Woman of Achievement award and the Jaycee's Outstanding Young Missouri Award. She is the Community Development Officer and Commercial Lending Officer for Premier Bank, Jefferson City, MO. Nancy is married to Bill Gratz and they have 3 children, 4 grand children, and 2 step grandchildren. She loves to spend time with her family, swim, and to play golf. ngratz@premierbank.com*

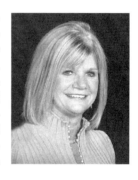

In August of 2001, Nancy Gratz was vice president of residential lending at a local bank. She almost canceled the appointment for her annual mammogram because she was very busy with new home loans and home refinancing at the time. Even though Nancy thought she felt a small lump just prior to her scheduled mammography, she briefly thought that it would be best to put off the exams until she first caught up with serving her clients at work. But her inner voice told her she needed to keep the appointment. Not only did she get her mammogram, but her intuition also nudged her to have additional diagnostic testing. A biopsy revealed Nancy had breast cancer.

"The doctor recommended a bilateral mastectomy. I was scared the day of the surgery because I didn't know how advanced the cancer was. I am very fortunate because it was detected early. I think what helped me to handle the diagnosis was being open to other survivors helping me and hearing what worked for them during their healing process. Plus I knew I wanted to be able to help other women in any way that I could after my survival," said Nancy.

"The most difficult part for me was staying strong around my family members and trying to be upbeat and positive all the time. Often I thought it was harder on them than it was on me. It was challenging for me to always keep a smile, but I prayed a lot for my health and for them. I reminded myself that cancer doesn't have me, and I believed I could get beyond breast cancer. I read a lot of inspirational books including *Chicken Soup for the Soul* books, *90 Minutes in Heaven* by Don Piper, *The Purpose Driven Life* by Rick Warren, and *Prescription for Life* because I thought these books would help me to stay strong and focused." said Nancy. "I admit that in my private moments, I did cry. And I did pray. My belief was that I was not going to let this get me, and that I was going to keep moving forward with my life and that is how I faced most days during my healing process. Things turned out positively, and I think this is because there were a lot of prayers."

At the time of diagnosis, Nancy was chairperson of the Chamber of Commerce in Jefferson City, Missouri. Because she couldn't raise her arms for a period of time after surgery, her husband Bill drove her to the executive committee meeting. She joked with everyone at the table about her new hairdo because Bill had to do her hair that morning. Nancy was determined that she was going to fulfill her duties and obligations as chairperson even though she was going through breast cancer. This helped her to keep a sense of normalcy in her life and was something she could have control of. She believes this determination and mindset, along with not isolating herself, helped her heal faster and to be able to return to work earlier than was medically expected.

"Since breast cancer, I do not spend as much time working but am spending more time with the people that I love. I live each day to the fullest, even though this sounds like a cliche', the little things have become so much more important to me. Things like cleaning my house isn't as important as it once was, but being with my grandchildren is. I have devoted more time to having fun. I knew I had to change my work situation, so that I would have less stress in my life because it was affecting my attitude. That is when I made the move to Premier Bank. I knew I had to slow down and my way of slowing down was to work in a place that I loved."

"I know that I am a stronger person as a result of living through breast cancer. My pledge is that if I can help some one in any way through their surgery and to help make their decisions easier, I will be there. The one thing that I can do is to share my experiences and try to help educate others. It is so very important. I have people thank me for helping them, even though it was some simple thing, but at the time you don't know how much it means to that person. I want to help women who are facing breast cancer as other people helped me. I encourage all breast cancer patients to connect with someone who has gone through the same experience. It makes the healing process so much easier. Always have hope and always share hope when you can. I believe that prayer also helped my emotional well-being along with my physical healing. Crying and laughter helped too. I want to thank my family, friends and other cancer survivors for the support they gave me to be able to say I am a 9 year cancer survivor. I also want women to know that their inner voice that speaks to take care of your health is a very important voice. Taking care of our health is so very very important," said Nancy.

Nancy Gratz is an amazing woman and her profile of wellness is exemplified in that she:
• Makes time for her health and healing needs in spite of busy work schedules
• Believes in intuition and the power of prayer
• Believes in healing possibilities
• Believes in fun, humor, and laughter in spite of being diagnosed with a life threatening disease
• Doesn't avoid her feelings and gives herself permission to cry
• Reflects upon her life and takes measures in her career so that she can enjoy her life more
• Expresses even more gratitude for her life, her family, and what is really important in life
• Believes in reaching out, receiving help, and helping others
• Believes in herself and others
• Believes in hope.

# 24.

# Thriving Beyond

## BY SHARON HENIFIN

*Sharon Henifin is the co-founder of Breast Friends, a non-profit organization that helps women survive the trauma of cancer. She is also a contributing author in GPS for Success: Goals and Proven Strategies, 2010. Sharon enjoys traveling, photography, reading, fishing, and camping with her husband and spending time with children, step-children, and grandchildren.*

*sharonhenifin@aol.com,*
*www.thrivingbeyond.com*
*mail@breastfriends.com*
*www.breastfriends.com*

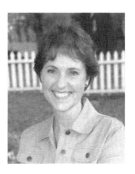

**B**ecoming a thriver didn't happen overnight, in fact, it took me several years and much heartache to move beyond feeling like a victim of breast cancer. It caught me at a time when I was already feeling down. Before the diagnosis I was dealing with the painful indiscretions of my husband at work, his dismissal from the company and all of the legal aftermath that ensued. It was a volatile marriage even before all of this happened, but I put up with it because I was raising our daughter and his two children that I loved like my own. We both worked for the same company so besides the humiliation, my career path came to a screeching halt.

My own identity was in question as I was adopted at ten days old and had hoped for many years to find my birth mother. After state records revealed my birth mother had used a fictitious name on my birth certificate, my chances of ever finding her looked dim. So in 1993 when I was diagnosed with breast cancer it seemed like I was being kicked when I was already down. But now, 17 years later, I can look back and see that there was a purpose in all of it. I can honestly say getting breast cancer was a blessing. It helped me discover the real "me."I'm doing work that is rewarding and makes a difference. I am married to a wonderful (different) man and I have taken control of my life and my happiness. I have strength I never knew I had. Because of breast cancer, I have become the woman I was designed to be and all the crazy ups and downs have made me stronger and resilient. And best of all, I've used my experience to help myself and others go the journey from victim to survivor, to thriver.

I found my own lump; it was a hard pea size nodule. Once I touched it, I knew in my gut I was in trouble. I called my doctor for that life changing appointment. Luckily I didn't have to wait long to get in to see my doctor. We exchanged all the normal pleasantries while being escorted to the examination room, but as soon as he had me lay down on the table, my heart was in my throat. I remember looking into his eyes for re-assurance and comfort. While his lips told me not to worry, his eyes screamed out the opposite. His warm brown eyes lovingly warned me, "This lump will change your life forever." At the time I didn't understand the enormity of what I saw in his eyes or what it meant to my future, but in time his message became crystal clear.

I had just turned 40 years old and was juggling work and family obligations when I found my cancer. I was the first person in my circle of friends to go through a life threatening diagnosis like breast cancer. I remember that navigating our health system felt like being on a sailboat alone and not knowing how to sail. I was at the mercy of the wind pitching me to and fro. My future was in the hands of doctors I didn't know or trust. I had six surgeries including a mastectomy with reconstruction and six months of chemo.

I remember looking at my diagnosis from a very scary place. Death and suffering had been my only association with cancer. When I started my journey, I feared that was may be my fate as well. I began to feel like a victim.

When I thought about my own mortality, panic took over. It was very disheartening to think I might not be there for my kids, or think someone else would raise them. I couldn't imagine not seeing my children graduate from high school or see them grow up and have their own families.

With life so uncertain, I found it necessary to compartmentalize my emotions just to get out of bed and get through each day. Most importantly, I had to try to keep my children's lives as normal as possible. I made a conscious decision not to expend any more energy on my mortality.

When the diagnosis was finally in, there was a glimmer of hope. The doctor had removed ten lymph nodes and fortunately none were cancerous. Armed with this one blessing, I was able to remind myself and my family that this was just a major inconvenience in our lives and we would get beyond this crazy roller coaster. We still had our moments of uncertainty because of the women we had known or heard of that had lost their lives to cancer. My youngest daughter's best friend had lost her mom to breast cancer, which of course, added to her fear as well as mine.

Though the prognosis was better than I expected, I still had to get through treatment. As if losing my breast, my hair, dignity, self esteem and self confidence wasn't enough, this life saving treatment caused immediate menopause. My tumor was fed by estrogen but at the time I couldn't believe how unfair it was to be thrown into menopause along with everything else I endured at age 40!

I recall my how my feelings of loneliness and isolation would sneak up on me. I looked horrible with my thinning hair, lopsided breast and pallid complexion. I didn't have the desire or the energy to put on makeup or even get dressed. I remember pushing myself to get off the couch and to take a short walk, or go to one of my kids activities; I knew down deep I needed to find my joy again. I'm a positive person by nature but during this time of healing and reflection I had to force myself to look for life's blessings.

It took me about a year to recover from the physical effects of cancer. I finally went back to work and tried to put the past year behind me. I stuffed many of my emotions deep down inside, trying not to worry about the cancer returning. My friends and family were thrilled when I finished my treatments and I could get back to normal. But I asked myself "Why didn't I feel normal? Instead of being glad my treatments were over, I was feeling even more terrified. I felt like I was no longer in the fight, but the enemy was lurking in every ache and pain. I was still in a battle, but this time without armor or weapons.

It wasn't until I began to share my experience with others facing the same battle that I truly began to heal emotionally. Over the years, I've learned that many women are private about their diagnosis, but from the beginning, I talked openly about my cancer experience. As time went on, I found myself answering questions from people asking me how they could help a friend or relative going through something similar. I was asked my opinion, told my story, but all those I spoke to were looking for one thing - hope. Even my plastic surgeon called me and asked if I would talk to some of his patients who were considering mastectomy and reconstructive surgery. I was always happy to speak to women or their families and share what I went through. Each time I shared, I found my burden being lifted just a little bit more. I realized it was energizing to share openly the details of my cancer.

In 1993, support groups were almost nonexistent. It wasn't that many years ago women wouldn't say breast or cancer out loud. Most still wouldn't talk about the emotional trauma that went along with the physical disfigurement. I started meeting the women referred by my doctor in a coffee shop or for lunch and realized quickly, I could answer most of their questions. I always got a kick out of the fact that the one question they wouldn't ask me was, "Can I see your reconstruction results?" They always wanted to know what it will look like after undergoing breast surgery, but they didn't want to impose. I found myself asking them directly "do you want to see what my reconstruction looks like?" After getting over their embarrassment, they jumped at the chance to see my results and were very thankful I offered. A look of relief immediately came over their faces and a sense of peace told me they could get through this just as I had.

I was continually amazed how sharing my results or even having a phone call with a total stranger made me feel better as well as it did them. It energized me to know I was making a difference in each one of these women's lives. It felt rewarding to share my story. I was able to empathize with their situation even if it wasn't identical to mine. All of our experiences are different, but there are enough similarities to allow us to bond. I referred many back to their doctors with questions they could ask or get clarification. The biggest thrill for me was to give each one of these women a glimmer of hope, a sense that if I had gotten through cancer, so could they. Each time I told my story I healed a little bit more. I was able to put the pain of my cancer experience behind me little by little by helping others cope with their emotions. In the process of sharing the most horrible time of my life I found my strength. I got a glimpse of what God put me on earth to do, and because of all of this, I started to thrive.

Three years after my initial diagnosis a very good friend of mine was told she had breast cancer. Unfortunately, Becky's cancer was more advanced and had gone into one of her lymph nodes. When I heard her news, I found myself crying, sobbing actually. I found myself crying more for her diagnosis than I did for my own. When I analyzed my strong reaction and the emotions I was feeling, I realized I was grieving my loss all over again. It reminded me again just how fragile life is, and how this disease still kills people. Since I understood what Becky was feeling, I found ways to support her through the next several scary and lonely months.

In 2000, Becky discovered yet another lump and we found ourselves waiting not so patiently, for her biopsy results. During those long daunting hours we spoke very frankly about why we both had survived this disease, and why we had remained friends all these years. We discussed the world of cancer and what we saw that was missing. Over lunch that day we decided that our experiences needed to be put to use. We agreed to start a non-profit organization dedicated to helping women survive the trauma of breast cancer...one friend at a time. We named it Breast Friends. Our firsthand experiences were the framework of our organization, using our knowledge of what kind of support a woman needs as she goes through cancer, and the ability to teach her friends and family how best to support her.

Both Becky & I had full time, high paying jobs with a large corporation that paid the bills, but it didn't take long to realize Breast Friends was our destiny. We spent all our available hours helping patients, creating the programs, raising money and everything that goes along with starting a nonprofit organization. Finally in 2006, I was able to retire from my corporate job and work full time doing what I loved. My identity was no longer split between what I did to make a pay check and what I did to make a difference. I could finally say with pride, "I am one of the co-founders of Breast Friends," knowing we are changing the lives of women and their families for the better.

We've done a lot of work in our local community, but in 2008 it became painfully obvious that survivorship issues were not being addressed after cancer treatment was finished. Cancer is a chronic disease in some cases; more patients are living longer than ever before. But with that, many women feel lost after their treatment, still dealing with side effects and unable to recapture their old selves. Their lives have changed forever, their self esteem and confidence have been brutally attacked, and "chemo brain" has made even getting a clear thought communicated more difficult. I understood what these women were going through, I had felt the same way myself but didn't know how to verbalize what I was feeling. So when I researched ways I could help these women find their footing again, life coaching stood out. I felt it was something I was meant to do and would simply enhance what I was already committed to.

After becoming certified as a life coach, I took the training materials and created a workshop for women to help them thrive. We discuss embracing their cancer experience and then ways to move beyond it and thrive. Many survivors suffer quietly with many issues, but during a "Thriving Beyond" workshop, these women have a safe place to talk about their lingering side effects, or their paralyzing fear their cancer may come back. They start to understand they aren't the only ones feeling as they do and, as the workshop progresses, they realize they are in charge of their future. I help survivors embrace what they have experienced, find the blessings, even the humorous aspects of their cancer, and help them create a plan to move forward.

It feels amazing to talk about matters that are significant and meaningful rather than shallow and trite. After looking at my mortality, I found power in me I never knew I had. I was able to realize an inner strength that has always been there, but I hadn't tapped into it till I took the focus off of myself and let it shine elsewhere. It was necessary to reach down deep into my character and learn to rely on my own strength and be the person I was designed to be.

My journey through breast cancer has allowed me to find my passion and, in turn, help others to find theirs. It has made it possible to get beyond old negative feelings, restore my spirit so I'm open to new adventures and repair weak aspects of my life. I was able to objectively assess and embrace the positive parts of my life and rid myself of the rest. Breast cancer has allowed me to discover who I really am, and what God put me on this earth to do. Breast Friends has become my vehicle to being the best I can be, thriving by sharing and caring for others. I have the opportunity to help others move from patient to survivor, and then to thriver.

Thriving comes by being able to focus on the positive, the dreams, and what really makes me unique. Life gave me the opportunity to evaluate what was going right, and what wasn't, and through my challenges encouraged me to make adjustments in my journey. I asked myself, "What brings me joy?" and then found ways to replicate those feelings in all areas of my life. I found working for a paycheck wasn't fulfilling, I needed to help others to feel good about myself. I learned to be grateful and focus on what I have, not what I was lacking.

I married a wonderful man; I have a great relationship with all of my children and have found my birthmother, four siblings and other extended family. I am traveling and creating many new adventures. There is life after cancer and I'm living it fully.

Passion makes life worth living. It's what makes us different, unique, and what makes us happy. When I think of something that I'm passionate about, it's no longer work, but fun. It actually creates energy. I can work a 12 hour day at something that I'm passionate about, and the time flies. I feel fulfilled instead of drained. Passion allows me to use my gifts and talents in a way that truly works. Discovering my passion has allowed me to thrive. Knowing my strengths and gifts has allowed me to find my passion, not my parent's passion or my teacher's or bosses'. It's an easy mistake to embrace someone else's dream instead of your own. I recently spoke with a lady who had worked in her family business for many years. She is going through treatment for a very aggressive cancer that has gone to her liver. We were enjoying lunch in a quaint outdoor bistro and I told her all about my life coaching and the workshop I had started. I inquired about her business and if it had been HER dream, she hung her head and admitted, "No, it was my husband's." I couldn't help but ask, "So what is your dream?" She straightened up and looked me right in the eye and said, "I don't know." The reality hit her that she wasn't living her dream; she was living someone else's.

I was fortunate. By being diagnosed at the age of 40, I was able to begin the journey of self-fulfillment at an early age. Some people wait their entire lives to figure it out. Don't make that mistake. Discover what your dream is now and take steps to make it happen. Find your passion and create goals around that dream. It will move you toward what's meaningful. Your life will be happier and more fulfilling. Find what you're really passionate about and make a difference in your surroundings and your community. You too will thrive.

None of us know how long we have on this earth. I had the opportunity to look at my own mortality and reflect on what is truly important in my life. It was a gift. Ask yourself, "What are my priorities?" "How do I want to leave this earth?" "What legacy do I want to leave behind?" Allow yourself to dream. As a teacher, Luzy Z. Martin once asked me, "What would you do if you knew you could not fail?" Discover your passion and thrive.

# 25.

# For the First Time In My Life, I Truly Felt Empowered!

## BY CHRIS HUBBARD

*Chris Hubbard has been a breast cancer thriver since 1995. She has a Masters Degree in Spiritual Psychology from the University of Santa Monica. She has been honored with the American Cancer Society's Theresa Lasser Award, and was listed as an Outstanding Young Woman of America for three consecutive years. Chris loves to participate in marathons and a woman's cancer survivor dragon boat team called The Pink Dragon Ladies. Her life coach practice, Four Rooms Life Coaching, provides assistance to others wanting to move from a place of fear, anxiety, and negativity during stressful situations toward a more positive and life-enriching approach by use of very creative action steps. She lives in Lutz Florida with her husband Barry and her working therapy dog, a chocolate lab named Rudy.*

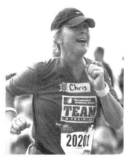

"Hum" I thought. "I've got a swollen gland in my breast. Oh well, it will probably go way in a few days." But, it didn't. So, after continually checking the lump for a few days, I thought it would be a good idea for a doctor to prescribe some antibiotics for my "swollen gland". After all, it couldn't be anything more serious than that. I wasn't concerned since I was only 42 years old with no family history of breast cancer, there had been no indication of any issues on the mammogram I'd had ten months earlier, and I was physically healthy in every other way. In fact, I was so confident there was nothing to worry about, I went to the appointment alone. After several needle biopsies and some hushed conversations, however, I began to get the feeling there was more to this lump than just a "swollen gland". I clearly remember—as it if were yesterday—saying to the pathologist and intern in the room with me looking at the biopsy slides, "So, what's the scoop, ladies?" The pathologist looked up from the slides and announced very matter-of-factly, "You have cancer." The stunned look on my must have given her the clue I was shocked because she quickly followed up with, "Well, you asked!" Before I knew it, I was scheduled for my first surgery instead of the antibiotics I was so certain would be prescribed.

My diagnosis was followed up with two surgeries, chemotherapy, radiation therapy, and Tamoxifen. Do I consider these treatments an element of my survival? Yes, no question about it. I believe my treatments were exactly what I needed to arrest the disease at that moment. In other words, the treatments provided by Western medicine afforded me the immediate intervention I needed to bring the cancer to a standstill. However, I also sensed my real long-term healing and prevention of occurrence would be contingent upon developing my mental, spiritual, emotional and physical needs to a new level.

Breast cancer provided an instantaneous wake up call. I understood I was being handed an opportunity to take an assessment of my life up to that point and a chance to make necessary changes to promote my own healing. For the first time in my life, I truly felt empowered. With this revelation, however, I also understood this new found empowerment would come with accountability. I realized I was responsible for the decisions and choices I had made up to that point—and those I would make in the future. This epiphany was both exhilarating and frightening at the same time. How does one go about taking an "assessment" like this? I decided the first step at each major aspect of my life: my mental, spiritual, emotional and physical way of being.

The physical inventory was relatively effortless. The obvious changes I could make in this area involved incorporating better dietary habits, prioritizing quality rest and adding exercise to my day. I will admit, however, the exercise piece was a little challenging. You see, I was always someone who avoided exercise at all costs. In the past, if there was a chance I was going to sweat, all activity would come to a halt. So, to thwart the tendency I had toward laziness, I committed to competing in a marathon. It didn't matter to me if I ran or walked or what my time was.... I just wanted to finish. This goal helped propel me out the door on a regular basis and, indeed, I did finish a full marathon!

My spiritual life had always been strong; I have always had faith in a Higher Power. However, facing a life threatening disease increased the importance of a spiritual practice into my daily life. I also began to see my relationship with God as a partnership. And, as with any partnership, a successful collaboration would require effort on my part. The final result was I decided to set aside time every morning to read uplifting material, pray and to write in my journal. I quickly discovered that as little as 10 to 15 minutes every day that I devoted to this was making a huge difference.

I began this exploratory journey by taking a blank sheet of paper and drawing a line down the middle. On the left side of the page, I listed all of the situations, experiences, and even people who had produced feelings of anger, resentment, anxiety or fear in me. The right side represented all of the situations, experiences, and even people who had produced opposite types of feelings. It was very easy to create a list for the left side (my "negative" side), however, I found there were very few items I could list on the right side (my "positive"side). I remember searching for a word to represent the right side of this document and the word that kept coming up was "joy". I actually had to look that word up in the dictionary to make sure I understood what it meant. I realized I was looking for something greater than just fun or enjoyment. I was looking for something closer to bliss. What I discovered from this simple exercise staggered me. I began to wonder if maybe my lifetime pattern of my negative emotional state had something to do with my diagnosis. Could years of being out of harmony have contributed to my illness? I read somewhere that prolonged stress might lower your immune system. Could this disease be a manifestation of my mental and emotional state? If there was even a kernel of truth to this, it was obvious I needed to remove as much as I could from the left/negative side of the sheet and I needed to add a lot more to the right/positive side. But, how could I go about doing this? Aha, how about a "Power Circle".

My "Power Circle" was an imaginary circle I drew around myself. I initially created this "circle" as a form of protection. By taking a hard look at my above-mentioned emotional inventory, I realized there were situations, experiences, and people I couldn't afford to have impact on me anymore, especially at this vulnerable time in my life. I imagined putting them outside my "circle". The only situations, experiences, and people I would allow inside my "circle" were those that brought me feelings of love, acceptance, support, or joy. For example, at the time, one of these people included my own mother. It's not that I didn't interact with my mother. I did. But, I instinctively knew she was not positively impacting my life, so outside the "circle" she went. I emotionally detached from her. I moved into an neutral emotional place when I had to have interactions with her.

Becoming more aware of my emotions, practicing detachment, and realizing I had the power to choose how I wanted to live my life was pivotal. Choice is a mental activity. Therefore, I decided my mental state would be greatly improved if I had a conscious decision about how I would react to, and feel about situations, experiences and people. I resolved to opt for forgiveness (forgiveness of myself and others), optimism (so much more pleasant than being full of "doom and gloom"), and laughter (nothing is more healing than a good belly laugh). I concluded I had allowed fear to prevail in my life. I made up my mind to eliminate as much fear from my life as I could. One way this was demonstrated was when I decided to make the effort to prioritize my needs. I had been raised to believe it was selfish to think of myself first. Imagine my shock when I realized I could take a walk instead of doing the laundry and my family wouldn't love me less or leave me. Another groundless fear dissolved!

In truth, this period of my life was one of the most joyous, peaceful, and enriching times I have ever lived through. When someone asked me to share my "story", I can only relate all the funny things that happened.... like the "sticky note" my husband put on my breast prior to my second surgery with instructions for the surgeon that said "Take what you need and leave the rest, and don't forget it's the right breast!" Or, the time I ran into two teenage boys while returning a video and having them announce their admiration for my "rad (bald) hairstyle." I am eternally grateful for the growth and learning I received as a result of this experience and if asked if I would do it again, I would definitely answer "yes". I am a better person for having had breast cancer and I know I have the power to keep this disease from appearing in my life again. You see, I've basically boiled things down to there are two emotions a person can choose to live their life by: fear or love. I choose love. What will you choose?

# 26.

# Choose Peace, not Fear

## BY SUZIE HUMPHREYS

*Suzie Humphreys is a much sought after motivational and inspirational speaker. She has been fired, been broke, been disappointed, been a petrified expectant mother at 40 years old and lives her life with a passion for learning not only how to be better, but to see things differently. She lifts, jolts and nurtures her audiences. She makes them laugh until they think they can't laugh anymore, and then she "grabs" them again. Her unshakable optimism in the goodness of life inspires each of us to better manage our own life experiences. Suzie is the author of If All Else Fails, Laugh. She makes her home in the hill country of Texas. www.suziehumphreys.com*

*It is never any good dwelling on what worries you. Fretting makes fear worse.*
*–Archie Moore*

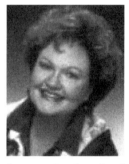

Well, the bad news is it's cancer. The good news is that it's at stage zero. "Okay! Right! Thank you for calling. No, I'm fine." I lied. "We'll go from here and just do what we have to do. Bye..."

"Okay, this is doable," I muttered, as I made my way to the office to tell my husband, Tom. Bracing myself to find the right words, I impulsively blurted out, "Honey, Dr. Diane called and I do have a little breast cancer. Now, before you say anything, I'm fine about this I really am. I mean if Christopher Reeves could go through paralysis and breathing on a respirator, I can do this. It could be so much worse." Tom just looked at me....partly stunned and confused at the same time.

"Suzie, a 'little breast cancer'? Is that like a 'little pregnant?' Sit down, please" he said. Then, taking my hands, he leaned across, and looking at me with those clear blue eyes said, "Well, here we are. If it's not this, then it might be that one of us slips and falls on the ice! It's just where we are at this stage in our life. We are going to get through this and you are going to be fine."

He was encouraging and he was right. I was going to do fine. After all, we decided to be fine there and then... piece of cake. Look at the calendar, I thought. You'll need to arrange your schedule and if you can just hold off on the surgery for two weeks, you can do the six speeches; cancel one, do the surgery on January 23 and be in Vegas on the sixth of February to speak to 900 dentists. It was as if I were starting rehearsals for a play. So, this was what it was like to face cancer. I hoped I would be brave. I could be an inspiration. Yes, that was the role I'd play. Like my friend Kay Russell who had double knee replacements, I would be the best patient my doctor ever had. The staff would all marvel at my good nature and my fearless determination to be an inspiration to those around me. That was the way I was going to play this life-drama out ~ a cross between Garbo's Camille and Doris Day's Calamity Jane. Poised yet perky.

There was to be a 'core biopsy'... something about which I knew nothing. I arrived at the scheduled time and half listened to the explanation of what the procedure involved. It would be similar to a mammogram only you lay down on your stomach on a padded table with a cutout where the breasts would hang down. Then, like a mammogram, the breast would be positioned so that very accurate pictures could be taken of the suspicious areas. Once those areas were pinpointed then a long yellow needle would be inserted by something akin to a 'staple gun' and sample tissue extracted. The needle was the easy part. The tough part was positioning and squeezing my breast.

Oh, nobody told me it would be like this. The pain came so suddenly it literally took my breath away, and then I started shaking uncontrollably and crying in great silent waves. I was so tense and in such pain I was frantically fighting to not tell them to stop. I was a baby, trembling and shaking until, in a matter of minutes, I was totally exhausted ~ and I let go. If you ask me what transpired in that cold examining room to that pathetic frightened "me" on that particular day, I would say "a miracle happened." And that "letting go" took me to the most peaceful, perfectly calm place that I had ever been in my life. Though the pressure was just as immense for the next several minutes and the pain just as intense, I didn't feel it. When I gave up my fight, I let go of the fear. The pain was still there, but I no longer felt it. My body and mind were just numb, as if I had crossed over the experience itself, still fully aware I was living it, but feeling disconnected from it. I remember thinking that crossing over the pain must be how mystics walk on beds of nails or burning coals.

Afterward, I told the doctors and nurses what had happened and how grateful I was to have had the whole experience. I had gone deeper and farther in what I call a "holy instant", an awareness of what our minds are capable of doing. I felt totally protected and loved and I knew without doubt that I was experiencing the "peace of God." I had always wanted to feel that experience. I had heard of others who had, but I never expected to find it, especially in the cold clutches of cancer. After I dressed and left the hospital to get into my car I remember being almost "out of focus".

I sat in the car and just cried hard and audibly, not caring if anyone in the parking lot could hear or see me. You know what I'm talking about don't you? You know how strong you can be in a crisis, fully functioning, thinking of everything that needs to be done, comforting others, preparing food, just busying yourself to stave off the reality of what really is happening inside you. And afterward, when the last guest has gone and the dishes cleaned, when the beds are turned down and everyone is tucked in, then maybe in a closet or some place out of reach from anyone interrupting....we just "let 'er rip." The tears just flow, the shoulders shake until the exhaustion comes and we slowly melt into the feather bed of peace.

I sat in the parking lot too dazed and numb to drive. And then totally alert, I remembered a prayer I had made to God. I have a special place on our ranch; a ten by twelve foot little cottage-like building that I call the potting shed. It serves as almost a "sanctuary" for me when I am tired, or troubled, or worried. It is like having my own church. I have a small iron bed in it, and a wonderful antique table filled with photographs of my family of loved ones, some still with us and some who have passed over. My special books are there, my soul books, my Bible, favorite art pieces I love, some crosses and candles that I burn in prayers for friends who are suffering or for strangers I see in the news that desperately need help and consoling. There are no sounds in the room, no air-conditioning motors, no telephones, no compressors, or buzzing from electric lines—just the rare sound of "silence."

It was almost a year earlier when I came home from a ten day trip and I literally could not wait to go to my little room "the potting shed". I was fatigued but happy, grateful to be home again and in my prayer of gratitude, I said to God in joy, "God, I don't want to leave this life without knowing all that you want me to learn. I am ready to learn it Father and I am willing to learn it any way you want to teach me." Sitting in my car after the "core biopsy", I wondered about "answered prayers." I wondered if I had subconsciously asked for cancer as my teacher. Certainly every time I met a cancer survivor, I had imagined what it was like for them to go through the treatments and hair loss and yet to joke about the turbans they wore or not having any eyebrows. Did I ask for this? Since it is a question to which there is no answer, I quickly knew that whether asked for or not, I was going to learn about what I was really made of. Whether I could take what lay ahead with humor and grace, or would I let my self down and those who loved me, by making it harder mentally than it had to be. If I could keep the "fear" at bay, I would do okay.

I called Kay from the parking lot and told her about the whole experience. She is one of four of my closest friends with whom I have been bound spiritually over the past twelve years. We are closer than sisters. We help each other through everything. We are gently honest with each other and we understand the depths to which we can descend in fear and the heights to which we can soar through faith. We have studied and learned and are joyful in our experiences. She cried with me on the phone and I went home to change my clothes and do a speech in the afternoon. The following day I was called by my doctor to tell me that we needed to do another core biopsy on the other breast. Well, I knew what to expect now, didn't I? I told Kay when I would be going and she wanted to come with me. I really do better if no one "hovers" over me, not that she would, but I get a lot of strength doing things by myself. I thanked her and told her how much I appreciated her concern and went on my way.

The following week, there I was again, lying in that cold room, on that cold padded table waiting for the "vise" to squeeze my good breast. Squeeze, it they did. But it was not at all painful. We all talked about how easy it was on me the second time, and during the chit chat my cell phone rang. I said, "I don't suppose this would be a good time for me to answer that?" The doctor replied from his little roll-around stool, "I don't suppose it would."

We went back to random chat, and in another fifteen minutes the procedure was ended. Still half dressed, but discreetly covered in a little teeny shoulder cape, I thought it would be a good time to check my cell phone message. After listening and laughing so hard, the nurses wanted to know what was so funny. So, replaying the message and putting it on speaker phone, they heard this message from Kay: "Oh Suzie, I feel horrible about what they are doing to you with that old core biopsy, I just can't stand it that you are in pain. I wish you had let me come with you but I know how independent you are and you are so brave. But if I could I would have gladly gone through this with you. I know you're probably out of there by now and I remember that you said you might be going to Neiman Marcus afterward and I was wondering if you were... would you mind stopping by the Bobbie Brown counter in cosmetics and pick me up a tube of lip-gloss!"

Oh how we laughed in that cold examining room. We laughed loud and hard and strong and all of us needed that, especially the nurses who, every day, deal with tragedy and with patients who come fearing the worse and hoping for the best. Kay certainly took me to that peaceful place again. I got there through a different form of transportation, but the results were the same. Peace with what was. Peace, whatever the circumstance. We are all walking around with an "it" of some sort. It can be cancer, or heart disease, grief over the loss of a loved one, a broken marriage, an estranged child, guilt over the past, or fear of the future. In each of the burdens is an opportunity to go beyond what we think we can do and flourish in the face of pain, despair and tragedy.

# 27.
# The Thriving Sisterhood

## BY LINDA JACKSON

*Linda Jackson is Founder and President of Ladies First Inc and Softee USA, and owner of Ladies First Choice, a breast cancer boutique in Salem, Oregon.*
*www.softeeusa.com*
*www.LadiesFirst.com*
*lindajackson@ladiesfirst.com*

Nothing could have prepared me for the shock of being diagnosed with breast cancer. At the age of 36 it was the last thing I thought would happen to me. I was completely uneducated about the disease, had no idea what to expect and was terrified to ask if I was going to die. It was an overwhelming and frightening time. Up until that summer day in 1985, I had always considered myself somewhat invincible; an independent, strong, resilient woman who could manage anything that life sent my way. For the first time, I felt completely vulnerable, alone and dependent on others for direction.

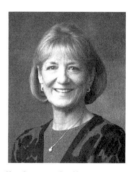

Upon hearing the news, my family and friends immediately rallied around offering concern and support which I greatly appreciated. I have no doubt that they did their best to understand what I was going through as they tried to reassure me that I was going be okay. But how could they possibly recognize or identify with my inner thoughts and fears or what it was that I needed, when I wasn't even aware myself.

Even though my prognosis was less than promising, from the beginning I was determined to overcome the cancer. I had three children to raise as well as aging parents who depended on me. I wanted to live and needed to believe it was possible to be healthy again. It was not easy to remain optimistic when I personally did not know of anyone who had survived breast cancer. Much later I would discover there were many, many women who went on to thrive following diagnosis and surgery—they were just not talking about it. In the 1980's breast cancer was still in the closet, a subject that women, especially those who were personally touched by the disease, did not openly discuss. At that time, there were also very limited, if any, resources available and no support groups specific to breast cancer. Unfortunately, it was an era of isolation for women like me who were searching for information and answers.

The bright spot in my recovery came when I found hope and inspiration from reading about actress Ann Jillian's battle with breast cancer. She was close to my age, diagnosed about the same time and was one of the first celebrities to go public with her diagnosis. She immediately became my hero. I admired her strong, warrior spirit and her decision to be openly candid about the details of her personal journey. Hearing her story helped me to understand that what one person chooses to share can make a positive difference in the lives of others.

Armed with the knowledge that overall healing can be found by connecting with a peer, a member of the "sisterhood", it became my mission to organize a breast cancer support group in my community. The focus was to create a welcoming, confidential place where women newly diagnosed, in recovery, those in treatment and veteran survivors could all gather to encourage each other and to face the challenges of survivorship together. I handed out flyers to the physicians in town, put up posters and advertised in the local newspaper. Much to my surprise, 34 courageous women attended that first meeting. There was an immediate connection as each person, some for the first time, began to share their personal stories of strength. Each was defined by a different background, diagnosis, surgery and treatment, yet in the end all of the stories were very much the same. The room buzzed with chatter about surgeries and treatments, prosthetic mishaps and hot flashes, followed by laughter as everyone understood and identified being on a common ground.

All of these years later the group is still going strong. Over time, the membership has changed as some women continue to stop by when they can, others take what they need then move on, while many choose to remain active to support the newly diagnosed. The success of this breast cancer support system is evident and is proof that we all have something meaningful to give or to receive by sharing what we each have learned.

I am grateful that today with breast cancer awareness and education in the forefront, no one has to face the journey alone as I once did. There are now breast cancer support groups in most cities around the country; resources and information available on the internet, in books and magazines. Many hospitals and breast centers offer patient navigators to educate and guide women from the time they are diagnosed, through surgery and into treatment. There are online support groups and national non-profit breast cancer organizations which provide 24 hour toll-free help lines as well as offer special programs to help those with financial need. Resources like these make it possible for women diagnosed with breast cancer today to have the knowledge and confidence needed to move forward to complete healing and wellness.

Since my initial diagnosis, I have had two recurrences—the most recent in 2004. I am thankful that, with the right treatments, both have been manageable. In many ways, having breast cancer has offered me many more positive life experiences than negative. My life has been more enriched as a result of the friendships and fellowship with other breast cancer survivors I have met along the way. I have learned it is okay to ask for help and to lean on others, to have faith in myself to make the right choices and to do the things I am most passionate about. I also discovered a whole new world I never would have known existed within the breast cancer community. It is here where I have found dedicated and caring healthcare professionals and hundreds of incredible survivors and thrivers who have chosen to share of themselves in order to serve and nurture others.

My doctors are perplexed and claim it is a downright miracle that I have survived this long. My Mother always told me I survived because I have important work to do. I don't know why I have survived this long beyond what modern medical experts thought I would, but I do know my life has been more enriched as a result of the fellowship of the breast cancer survivors and thrivers that I have met and how I have gleaned on their experiences of strength and fortitude and compassion.

# 28.

# I Am a Thriver!
# I Am Vigilant About My Health

## BY VALERIE JACKSON

*Chief Master Sergeant Valerie D. Jackson is from Reading, Pennsylvania and graduated from Reading High School in 1977. She enlisted in the United States Air Force as an Administrative Specialist on April 24, 1978. She has a Masters Degree in Public Administration Management and Bachelors Degree in Business Management. In 1982, as a talented vocalist, she was selected for the United States Air Force Academy Band in Colorado Springs, Colorado. Her entertainment highlights were sharing the stage with Wayne Newton at Caesar's Palace in Las Vegas, Nevada and Neil Sedaka at the New Orleans Worlds Fair in Louisiana. She also sang with gospel recording artist, director and composer Reverend Milton Biggham at Osan Air Base, Korea and Vanessa Williams at her church in Maryland. In 1986, she returned to the administrative career field. Her background includes various duties in administration, protocol, entertainment, security, information management, passport processing, operations, personnel management, education and training for officers and senior executive service members and enlisted counseling. She served her country for over 29 years and retired on March 1, 2007. vjackson66@aol.com*

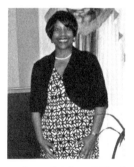

I served over 29 years in the United States Air Force, but the hardest battle I had to fight was breast cancer. Ironically, the "fighting" part of breast cancer was not the most difficult challenge. It was dealing with hospital administrators, physicians, schedulers, and technicians in determining the proper treatment for the breast cancer.

I quickly learned I had to be my own advocate for my health. No one knows my body better than I. I felt a lump, it didn't feel right and I experienced pain. The lump was not identified on my mammogram or ultrasound. My military physician told me, "I didn't have cancer because I didn't fit the profile, I didn't smoke or drink and I had no family history of cancer." Additionally, he said it was probably a fibroadenoma and that cancer doesn't hurt.

After several hospital visits on this matter, I finally met a doctor who referred me to the National Navy Medical Center's Breast Care Center. The doctor felt the golf ball size lump, did a fine needle aspiration and scheduled me for surgery the next day. This is just one example of my "fight" with cancer, that it took several visits to be properly tested. (So much for early detection.)

Another misdiagnosed experience was in August 2004, six months after my last radiation treatment. I notified my doctor that I had a bloody discharge from my right nipple.

For three weeks, the doctor kept telling me it was residual from having radiation. I told the doctor I was tired of driving 70 miles to be told the discharge was residual from radiation. I suggested he at least do a blood culture to determine the problem. The doctor told me "If that will make you feel better, I'll do it, but I've seen this discharge in several of my patients. It's nothing to worry about." The doctor called me the next day and said I still had cancerous cells in my breast. When I later visited the doctor, he wanted to remove both of my breasts because I was top-heavy and said I'd be lop-sided if he removed only one breast. Needless to say, I demanded a second and third opinion and transferred my care to Johns Hopkins Medical Center.

I found the first alarming lump in my right breast in 2003. Six weeks after radiation in 2004, I informed my doctor about a bloody discharge in my right nipple. Four years later I found another lump in 2008 and had chemo and radiation in 2009. Consequently, I've had 13 cancer related surgeries. Through this experience, I have learned to be vigilant about my health. I've written letters to hospital commanders telling them my experience. I emphasized not everything is written in black and white. The letters were not to reprimand the hospital staff, they were written to improve the hospital process. At times, I felt alone because no one thoroughly examined me or addressed my concerns. No one should go through cancer alone. I often mentioned cancer wasn't killing me, the administrative bureaucracy was.

I believe my vigilance for my well being has changed my life for the better since having breast cancer. I retired from the military and I now travel to spend quality time with my family and friends. Before retirement, I was always worried about things that were not as important. Poet/Writer Emily Matthews eloquently stated, "It's not what we own or buy that signifies our wealth, it's the little things that have no price - our family, friends and health." The people I cherish and things I value the most are my family, friends and my health.

I visit my family more. I see my nieces and nephews grow into young adults versus hearing their reports by phone or e-mail. I'm setting a good example for my relatives and friends by returning to school for another Masters degree. I want to continue being a role model for the young and old. I can still smile and say, "I've made it after all I've gone through." The role I played in making changes for the better started with my choice and desire to live. I'm a Thriver and a 3x Cancer Survivor.

I empowered myself to help others dealing with cancer to choose to live. I help their spiritual growth through my personal testimonies of God's goodness. I encourage others to improve their health through exercise, change of diet, massage therapy and to surround themselves with positive people to help their healing process. By enhancing and encouraging others, I'm increasing their knowledge of cancer and enhancing their confidence and their will to live. That's what being more vigilant about life is about.

One of the most important lessons in my healing experience was to know that being diagnosed with breast cancer was not my death sentence. The struggle was to really believe this, especially when my greatest fear was of dying alone while away from my family. I kept reminding myself and my family members that in life and in death I am never alone because I am a child of God's.

As a spiritual person, I relied on God's grace and mercy that I am healed. Philippians

3:4 says "I can do all things through Christ which strengthens me." I prayed for my healing and asked others to pray for me. Also the many cards, calls and visits from family, friends and church members touched my life and helped my healing process.

Laughter was another healing tool. I had a sense of humor about having cancer and kept others laughing. Sometimes people feel sorry for or pity cancer patients. They don't know what to say or do. When I make people laugh I put them at ease and take their focus off of my temporary condition. I told one relative to stop leaving me depressing messages on the phone as if I was on my death bed. I told him I've got the Victory and I was on my way to a full recovery!

I talked with elderly cancer survivors at my church. Seeing and talking with them gave me hope that I too would make it. Those folks had cancer 20-30 years ago when more drastic measures were taken and they're still alive. That's a testimony.

I learned that it is one thing to survive, but in order for me to thrive, I had to take care of myself first and to make my health and well-being the number one priority in my life was vital. I take time to share my experiences with others to preclude them from going through the same situations.

I learned to be vigilant about my health and I use these ten principles still today.

1. Because proper sleep is so important for my body to restore itself, I made sure I got proper rest. I set boundaries to make sure I was able to sleep well.

2. I followed up on any concerns in my body. I obtained second and third opinions.

3. I changed doctors when I wasn't comfortable with the information they provided me with or if they were not attentive to my health needs.

4. I removed myself from family drama. I stopped driving home every time there was a family crisis and I focused on what I needed in order to heal.

5. I never considered myself a victim and I didn't allow others to consider me one. Even though I was shocked when I was first diagnosed with breast cancer, I was thankful that I didn't have a military deployment at that time.

6. I surrounded myself with positive and encouraging people.

7. I exercised to keep up my strength and energy.

8. I had a monthly massage and practiced the Reiki Principle. To Heal-thy-Self equates to a healthy self through meditation and visualization.

9. I gave to others and I learned to make something greater in my life as a result of the breast cancer experience. When life presents you with a lemon, we know we are to make lemonade. As a three time cancer survivor, I've lectured and shared my story with young Soldiers, Sailors, Airmen and Marines in the military. I've joined the cancer ministry at

my church. I continually help other cancer patients through their journey. I'm known as the Thriver with the warm heart and big smile. I'm a walking testimony that healing is possible. I provide others with information on cancer. I drive patients to chemo/radiation therapy. I listen and answer questions that patients have about cancer to ease their anxiety. I take cruises, workout and attend massage therapy classes. At church, we're in the process of establishing a mini command-post to assist church members that need support, information or transportation to their cancer appointments.

10.  Finally, anything to improve the process is what I share with hospitals, administrators and advocators of cancer wellness. I am vigilant about my health by sharing my experience with others. If I can help someone by sharing my story, I'm going to tell it!

# 29.
# Be a Thriver! I Love That Statement

## BY HEATHER JOSE

*Heather Jose was diagnosed with stage IV breast cancer at 26. She chose to fight the cancer head on by putting together a plan to battle cancer on a daily basis. Eleven years later, Heather is healthy and using her experiences to speak to healthcare providers and patients about how much their words and actions can impact success. Heather is the author of "Letters to Sydney; Every Day I am Killing Cancer." www.heatherhose.com*

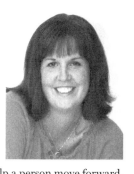

Be a thriver! I love that statement. It implies action and an attitude of gratefulness. It says that how we approach things matter. I know that is true. Each one of us can make a difference in our health and wellness.

Cancer is a funny thing. It can bring out the best and the worst in people. It really depends on how you approach it. Now, that is not to say that those that approach it with an attitude of thriving rather than surviving live rather than die. But those that thrive really live, no matter how many days they are in this world. And guess what? We are all going to die, so my goal is to make the most of my days. Acknowledging death might even help a person move forward.

I believe that everyone can learn to thrive through cancer. I also believe that it may take a major adjustment in the way we view our world. But the rewards are great, a life of purpose, one lived with eyes wide open to the wonder of each day.

In the first letter that I sent to my family and friends to tell them about the challenge of cancer I said, "We are not saying why me, rather we are saying try me!" You could say that was me being young and dumb at the ripe old age of 26, but it set the tone from the start. I knew that I was going to do everything I could to kill the cancer and live the best life possible. My intuition told me that I needed to find out what I could control and do that, because it made me feel better. I also felt deeply that focusing on the extremely dreary statistics was exhausting and could negate the best things that I had done for myself each day.

I have spent a lot of time thinking and writing about what makes some women thrive while others stay in survival mode. It is not a formula that you can plug in for each person or something that you can bottle and disperse. Thrivers take their strengths and build on them. They acknowledge their weaknesses and let them go. Thrivers are willing participants in their own health, they are not waiting for someone else to fix them. I chose to work closely with my medical team, because I am in charge of my body. Thriving is a process of taking in information and using the very best of it to keep moving forward. This does not mean getting bogged down in the endless info, which can capture our minds in a negative manner. It is continual growth, recognizing that part of that process is in nurturing one-self and resting when needed. Thriving is greeting each day with a spirit of making good choices and living fully.

Let's take a look at survival for a minute. When diagnosed, we immediately become survivors. I thought I would look up the definition for that.

sur·vive *v.*
*sur·vived, sur·viv·ing, sur·vives*
1. To remain alive or in existence.
2. To carry on despite hardships or trauma; persevere
3. To remain functional or usable

survivor *n.*
1. a person or thing that survives

This is not how I want to be described, ever. Because I believe that there is so much more in life than just survive. There are moments in life that I survived, yes, but to simply remain alive or in existence? No thanks.

thrive *(thr v)*
*intr.v. thrived or throve (thr v), thrived or thriv·en (thr v n), thriv·ing, thrives*
1. To make steady progress; prosper.
2. To grow vigorously; flourish:

Thriving is about attitude. I was once talking with a woman about the changes that I had made in my diet in relation to cancer. Her response to me was very telling.

"Don't you ever just want to have a chocolate chip cookie?" she implored.

"If I want a cookie, I will have one and move on," I told her, "but most of the time, I would choose a life watching my kids grow over a cookie."

Her statement showed me that she was not embracing the attitude of a thriver. I don't feel restricted because I have made dietary changes, I feel empowered that I can make a difference. I don't feel guilty when I stray from my diet, I simply try again tomorrow. When I workout, I focus on how good it is for my body, not how much it hurts. Likewise, I asked not to know the side effects of medications or the spots of my bone mets, so that I would not focus on them. (My husband knew them, just in case.) I know that the head games are just as significant as the physical impact of my choices. We are physical, mental and spiritual beings and we have to address each of these aspects to thrive. It is our own unique makeup, however, as to the order in which we address them.

Bev Vote and I were talking about this order recently and laughing about how different we are. For Bev, I would list her as spiritual, mental and physical where as I am the complete opposite. What we have in common is belief that we impact our bodies with our thoughts and actions and also more than a normal amount of determination (or some might call it stubbornness). Regardless of the order or the way we approach a life without cancer, we both believe it can be done.

Because of the impact of cancer in my life, a million good things have happened. It has helped me to focus on the positive and believe that anything is possible. It has confirmed my belief in God. It has shown me that family is not a right, but a gift, and that families are built in a lot of different ways. I have learned not to take my body for granted. It has helped me want to make the most of each day. It has revealed my passion for life.

I am a woman. A wife. A mom. A daughter. A friend. I am a writer and speaker. And yes, I sat in a doctor's office one day and listened as he told me to 'get my affairs in order' because I had breast cancer. That was a life changing day, no doubt, because it started me on the path to my real life, the life that I believe I was created to live.

Life is full of choices. Thriving through adversity is one of them.

# 30.
# Writing in Search of Wellness

## BY BEVERLY KIRKHART

*Beverly Kirkhart is a breast cancer thriver and author of My Healing Companion and
co-author of My Healing Companion: A Journal for the Health Care Provider and Chicken
Soup for the Surviving Soul: 101 Healing Stories About Those Who Have Survived Cancer
Beverly is a trained, certified journal-writing instructor. She has been heard by millions
across the country as a featured inspiration keynote speaker and journal workshop leader
for top organizations, cancer hospitals, non-profit groups, and medical centers. In 1996, she
co-founded the highly regarded Breast Cancer Resource Center of Santa Barbara. Beverly
resides in San Luis Obispo, California, where she is Director of the Hearst Cancer Resource
Center. Her work allows her to continue to devote her life to helping patients everywhere to
take control of their lives, and turn their setbacks into comebacks. www.beverlykirkhart.com*

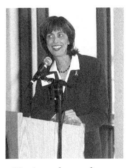

I was living the American dream. Married to my college sweetheart, together over our seventeen years of marriage we designed and built our dream home. We also owned and operated an eighteen-room bed and breakfast, just eighty-four steps from the Pacific Ocean. I loved my life! But in 1991, this dream life shattered. My marriage ended in a divorce. Then, only months later, I lost the business and home that I thought I would have for the rest of my life. I found myself standing in the unemployment line. If that wasn't enough hardship, in 1993 I heard my doctor say, "Beverly, you have breast cancer."

What immediately followed was a whirlwind of confusion. Having always been a healthy person with little experience in the medical world, I found myself overwhelmed and frozen with fear when receiving my cancer diagnosis. I was intimidated by the medical system and uncertain about what questions to ask, who to see and why. Where do I go, who do I turn to? Can someone help me with these unfamiliar frightening feelings of anger, despair, and betrayal?

My world was turned upside down. I desperately needed to share my feelings and emotions. But, confused and scared, I considered being the "perfect patient" and not bother my medical team or loved ones with my deepest fears and concerns. I thought to myself, Keep your mouth closed and do as you are told. Buck-up, be strong, and don't reveal your emotions. This is exactly what I did. I simply did not share.

Keeping my feelings to myself was normal for me. Most of my life I had been someone who did not easily express my thoughts or emotions for fear of being judged or criticized. But when cancer came into my world, I had a flood of frightening and unfamiliar feelings that consumed me. I had no skills or knowledge of how to verbalize these negative, terrifying thoughts. Instead, I pushed them aside or buried them deep inside. In choosing not to address these issues, I found myself feeling miserable, depressed and extremely pessimistic. Eventually these ugly buried feelings began to take a toll on my physical health and emotional well-being.

How we choose to look at our situation has a direct affect on the outcome. If we elect to be consumed by our negative thoughts it can affect our healing process.

The role of the patient's attitude during cancer treatment has been debated for years. There are many who believe that having a positive attitude does not have an affect on long term cancer survival. But most physicians, researchers, psychologists and oncology specialists strongly support the idea that cancer patients who have an optimistic attitude will have a higher tolerance to their treatments.

Hearing a cancer diagnosis for most patients stirs up a hurricane of emotions– anger, despair, betrayal, deep sadness, and fear. There is no right or wrong way to respond to a cancer diagnosis. We are all unique; one of a kind. Each of us reacts differently to bad news. It is okay to feel angry or frightened. It is okay to feel like a victim, betrayed or despair. But we can't stay stuck in these negative feelings. It is critical to our health that we don't stay angry or feel like a victim for a long period of time. We need to find healthy ways to express and let go of our emotions.

I found journaling to be my method of coping with my deep feelings. It allowed me to move beyond my negative, physically and mentally destructive thoughts to stay strong and upbeat during challenging times.

I discovered journaling at the beginning of my treatments. My nurse suggested I consider expressive writing as a way to release my thoughts and feelings. She explained it would be valuable for me to have a voice to express my fear, anger, and sadness. Perhaps I had a voice that wasn't verbally strong, but on paper she said it would roar! Reluctant and a little resistant, I opened a blank journal and began writing out my thoughts and fears. This wasn't easy for me at first because I'm dyslexic and a poor speller. I avoided writing like the plague. But with encouragement from my nurse, I let go of the fear and self-judgment and allowed the words to flow out on paper. As I freely wrote, I began to understand more clearly why I felt the way I did. As a result of my daily writing, I came to realize I wasn't a cancer "victim", but rather an individual with God-given gifts!

Journaling helps us clean out the negative thoughts that occupy and take up space in our brain. It frees the mind to be creative, solve problems and can give insight into the causes and cures of a difficult challenge. Journaling was so valuable for me that I wanted to share it with others. I took excerpts from my journal, and put them into a hard bound book I call *My Healing Companion*. Released in 2001 with 150,000 copies in circulation, this is a self-directed journal to help the patient find emotional healing through writing.

There is increasing evidence to support the notion that journaling has a positive impact on our physical well-being. University of Texas at Austin psychologist and researcher James Pennebaker, who is a pioneer in the study of using expressive writing as a route to healing, contends that regular journaling strengthens the immune cells.

Clinical studies at MD Anderson showed that cancer patients who repeatedly recorded their thoughts experienced increased vigor, sounder sleep and reduced stress. Annette Stranton, PhD, designed a study at the University of Kansas in Lawrence with 60 women who had early-stage breast cancer. Those who expressed their deepest thoughts and feelings reported significantly decreased physical symptoms. The group who wrote positive thoughts and feelings regarding their experience had significantly fewer medical appointments for cancer-related morbidities.

Journaling studies continue to confirm what many cancer patients know, and what I certainly have experienced, writing down your deepest thoughts and feelings may improve the quality of life for a cancer patient.

I remember in 1993 when I heard "Beverly, you have cancer." It was the final tragedy in a series of tragedies that had led me deep into despair. I swam in a sea of negativity, anger and of mental and physical anguish. It wasn't easy, but I learned to appreciate myself and my gifts.

I discovered that journaling helped me to see the best in me, and I want that for you, too! I encourage you to give journaling a try—what do you have to lose? You have so much more to gain. The pen is waiting for you to let the words flow out on paper. Go ahead....let your inner beauty and strength come through your written words and begin to see the gifts you have offer to the world.

If you've never kept a journal, here are some tips to get you started...

1. Date every entry. This will help you to create a benchmark of your progress. Also, chronologically it will provide you with reference points along your journey.

2. Find the specific time of the day that best works for you. Don't let anything but emergencies interfere or pull you away. Also, don't say "no" to an urge to write at anytime. Give yourself the freedom to jot down your thoughts whenever they occur.

3. Find a place to write that is comfortable, relaxing and peaceful. Perhaps it's a room in your house, or your patio, or the library, or your favorite coffee shop.

4. Privacy versus sharing. If you don't want people to read your journal, find a secret place to store it or write across the front "Private." Consider telling those who might be tempted to read your journal that the journal is not for their eyes. You won't feel the freedom to write honestly if you are concerned someone will read it. However, if you do feel like sharing, please do so - this is empowering for you and the reader.

5. If you decide to write at home, create a stimulating environment. What moves you? Is it music? Burning candles? The aroma of a cup of tea or espresso? For me, it was turning on a soothing tape and writing by candle light.

6. What to write in? If you don't have a copy of *My Healing Companion*, think about investing in one of the bound journals now available at many bookstores or stationary departments. If a thought occurs when your journal isn't available, grab a piece of paper or napkin, and write!

7. Give yourself permission to write any way you want. Now that you have all your writing tools, where do you start? Make a list of your emotions. To unleash these emotions, pick a word, feeling or quote. If you're happy, consider writing in pink ink. If you're sad, try blue ink. Also, write big, write small, from left to right, in a circle, whatever your mood dictates. If you can't find the words, draw a picture. Let the child in you roam free and your spirits will follow.

8. Don't edit yourself. We already spend too much time judging ourselves. Trusting yourself means giving your feelings full-rein to come out. Who is going to care if you misspell a word or don't write complete sentences! It's your journal, and no one will ever see it—unless you want them to.

# 31.

# What We Decide To Do With These Circumstances Makes Us Who We Are

## BY LORI LOBER

*Lori Lober's personal brush with cancer came in 1998 when she found a suspicious lump in her breast. A doctor's visit revealed that the lump was a non-cancerous fibrocystic disease. In 2000, after feeling increasingly ill since her examination two years earlier, Lori went to another doctor. This time, she was a stage four breast cancer patient and the disease had metastasized to her liver. Lori was diagnosed with an estimated 12-18 months to live. Traditional cancer treatments at that time offered little hope of long-term survival. The odds she would even be alive five years later were less than 3 percent. After extensive research, Lori created an integrative treatment plan incorporating the best of Western conventional medicine with complimentary therapies. This research also led her to a Comprehensive Cancer Center with an innovative team of doctors and a clinical trial that included a biological therapy that attacked her cancer cells while leaving her healthy cells unharmed. Her tumors responded well to treatment and now, more than ten years later, there is no evidence of the disease in her body. The life-altering experience left Lori deeply touched by the support she received from her husband, friends and family, inspiring her to form the Touched by Cancer Foundation and to help and to give hope to others. Her second book, "Still Bigger than Pink: Alive and Thriving!" includes her personal journeys of combining both Eastern and Western medicine. Lori continues to thrive and has been an active advocate for integrative care, biotechnology, clinical trials, and optimal health and wellness through nutrition. She and her husband John live in Kansas City, MO with their rescued kitty cats, Lucky and Cosmo, Bon Jovi, Daughtry, Nickelback, and their black lab, Grace. www.BiggerThanPink.org / www.WeLovetoLive.com*

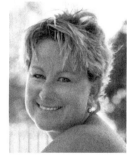

Fear... Disbelief... Blame—April, 2000—MY WORLD WAS CRUMBLING—it would never be the same, as I knew it.

But now, OVER TEN YEARS LATER—I feel as though my stage four, metastatic breast cancer diagnosis was a gift from God!

How & why can I feel this way?! Keep reading!

Today, August 1, 2010—a bright, happy sunshine-filled Sunday in Kansas City, MO! Still, after everything I have been through over the course of the last ten years, I feel truly blessed. Not only am I surviving, I AM THRIVING!

Each of us faces turmoil, setbacks and challenges throughout our lifetime. It is truly what we decide to do with these circumstances that makes us who we are.

I remember, immediately after my diagnosis, Sister Alice Potts at M.D. Anderson Cancer Center told me that even though I was facing the fight of my life, CANCER WOULD

NOT DEFINE WHO I WAS AS A PERSON UNLESS I ALLOWED IT TO. She was right in so many ways and I will thank her forever for giving me that expert advice!

I was very happily married to John Lober and had been for a long time. I was content in my life. We were home builders and had achieved much success in the industry. For this I am grateful—but, for the success attained we paid a price—it was a very fast-paced, activity-filled lifestyle. We were always expected to attend events, galas, parties and too many social gatherings to mention.

So many, in fact, that I feel my cancer was feeding itself because of a compromised immune system—not enough rest, not eating the right foods, not enough self-love. Instead I was trying desperately to be the person everyone thought I should be.

Cancer was a gift to me because I was able to step back from what was expected of me—I was able to focus on myself for the first time, probably ever. I was able to embrace the best treatments Western medicine had to offer! I was able to integrate meditation, receive acupuncture, reflexology, therapeutic massage, chiropractic care—things I had never experienced "BEFORE CANCER". I understood that what I was fueling my body with, an acid-rich environment, was also fueling my cancer.

My cancer diagnosis was also a blessing because it has brought so many beautiful people into my life that I know, without my diagnosis, I would have never met. The reverse is also true. Cancer allowed me to rid myself of negative people in my life—I felt lighter immediately!

John, my only child, Colby and I were able to start checking off items on our bucket list—what a blessing! How often does any other 36-year old get to start working on her bucket list? I was making memories, taking photos and making scrapbooks for Colby and John! I wanted them to remember me after I died.

Why did I have to be diagnosed with the worst and final stage of cancer in order to understand the importance of taking care of myself and my health? I often wonder this but instead of worrying about it I use my life lessons to help others who hear the dreaded words "you have cancer". That was my promise and I am proud, ten years later to say that I am alive and well, am "NO EVIDENCE OF DISEASE" and fulfilling all of the promises I made to God for keeping me alive and well. I feel I am healthier now then I've ever been in my life—both inside and outside, mentally, physically and emotionally!

How can this be? In my opinion, a cancer diagnosis is a huge wake up call. We can make changes, embrace whatever treatment we feel is best for us, see ourselves as whole and well on the other side of the cancer journey OR we can succumb to it and ultimately die.

This too, may be a gift—just think about others who pass away with no notice—no time to say goodbyes to loved ones, no time to get their affairs in order, to distribute coveted collections, china or jewelry to loved ones. Cancer, if seen like this, can be a gift to everyone who is diagnosed with it.

Why do I say this? Because I was not able to say goodbye to my only child. You see, when I was diagnosed with cancer, I prayed that I would see Colby graduate from high school—he was 13 at the time and all odds were against me. (At stage four I only had a 2% chance of being alive for five years.)

But, I saw it in my mind—I saw me watching him walk across the stage and receiving his high school diploma. What I didn't see is what would happen next.

On a gloomy Monday morning, on icy roads in Kansas City, MO, I would lose my only child in a horrific car accident. He had been accepted into the coveted 6-year medical school program at UMKC. He was loved by everyone who knew him and life as we lived it then was amazing and beautiful.

In one quick moment, things as we know them can change. The memories, the photos and the scrapbooks I had been making during my cancer treatments were for me. They were for me to remember the beautiful moments I was able to share with my son; before HE went to Heaven.

I could have played the victim card. Who would that help? It wouldn't bring Colby back. It would make John and my friends miserable and I, too, would be a depressed and miserable person. Instead, I chose to do the same thing I did when I was diagnosed with final stage breast cancer. I chose to see the 19 years and 1 week I WAS ABLE TO SHARE with my son as a gift. I believe the five years, after my cancer diagnosis I was able to spend with Colby working on our bucket lists was a gift that can never be taken away from me.

Now I challenge you—if you are reading this book, you or someone you love either has cancer or has had cancer. Maybe you're supposed to share one or more of these stories with others who need to be inspired to live, to do something positive with their cancer diagnosis, or possibly even embrace their cancer journey and make the best of the final days, months or years of their life.

Take an active role in your journey, ALWAYS ASK FOR MORE THAN YOU THINK YOU WANT and most importantly, choose to be happy, choose to be healthy and choose to love and be loved!

# 32.

# Becoming Amazon

## BY ROBYN LYNN

*Robyn Lynn had no risk factors when she was diagnosed suddenly with breast cancer in 2008 at the age of 39. She is mom to Megan, 21 and Eric, 18, and lives with her partner Neil and their 3 chickens in the Seattle area. Robyn writes a blog about the warrior lessons learned on the path to wholeness and in her spare time manages a ski shop. She is a local and national Reach to Recovery volunteer with The American Cancer Society and can be reached at becomingamazon@gmail.com or visit her blog: http://becomingamazon.com.*

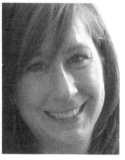

One summer evening finds me in the uncomfortable position of being the focus of attention as I stand in the center of the large group of gathered women. It is dusk, the wind is dying down and the swallows have begun to dip and dive around the meadow. Heat from the day radiates from the ground under my booted feet but I am covered in goose-bumps. A forgotten fire in the pit next to the gathered women smokes and pops. The sudden snap of the banners planted in the ground in each of the four directions makes me flinch. Wearing my work clothes from the lodge fire I have been tending for the past 4 days, I am closely surrounded by a dozen or so women wearing versions of "warrior" costuming ranging from full on Middle Ages chainmail to Amazonian/Xena fantasy. Stuffing my leather gloves in my back pocket I remove my denim shirt to catcalls that immediately fall silent. I walk to the front of the group wearing only my dirty jeans and work boots. All eyes are on me. I am bare-chested standing in front of 150 suddenly silent and crying women and the smooth plane and deep scar where there used to be a right breast cannot be ignored. I raise my makeshift homemade bow to the sky and pull back the string aiming for the newly emerging stars and tears begin streaming down my face.

~ ~ ~

About a year after my journey with cancer I was attending a Women's Summer Solstice retreat in eastern Washington with my then 20 year old daughter Megan. This has been an annual event for us—one that appeals much more to her bohemian theatrical self than to my own quieter earth based spiritual side. But I have found my place as one of the leaders of the Lodge community—a small group of women who hold ceremonial and prayer space for the gathering through the use of a Native American inspired sweat lodge that is open to the participants. My role leaves me well known at the gathering, but I have only a passing, albeit meaningful, connection with most of the women. Only a handful knew how I had spent the past year.

As a part of the gathering, women have the opportunity to lay claim to one of many offered archetypes (Maiden, Mother, Crone... etc.) to celebrate attributes that they are recognizing now or would like to manifest . It is a public statement of sisterhood and commitment to a path of growth in a certain area. The way of Amazon—or woman warrior—is one of the offered archetypes representing the qualities of female strength, power, leadership and triumph over challenges. The legendary female tribe of Amazon warriors were respected as ferocious, courageous fighters who reportedly cut off their right breast as young girls in order to allow them to pull a bow sting unhindered. Symbolically at this gathering women claim Amazon relating to the warrior spirit and the idea of having had to "sacrifice" pieces of themselves in order to bring out their inner strength.

Years prior to this, I had claimed the path of Amazon in celebration of being an abuse survivor - an honoring of the strengths I gained through adversity and a commitment to being a leader within my community. This year, following my full, right sided mastectomy, the irony of reclaiming Amazon couldn't be ignored. My good friend Carole, also a recent breast cancer survivor with a right side mastectomy, decided that now was the time to claim our right to acknowledgement for the challenges we have faced. Surrounded by the love of our friends, teachers and family and many total strangers we made this a time of honoring the more private parts of our path that are nevertheless a shared theme among all women..

The claiming of my own body—claiming the scars that are a testament to my strength and a diary of the trials that I have been through was the driving force behind my decision to bare my chest in front of so many people who would have otherwise never known what I looked like under my shirt. As a 40 something, reasonably good looking, fit, unmarried mom, this was a claiming of my body as attractive in a world that judges "attractiveness" by plastic surgery, enhancements, push up bras and air-brushing. Here was the bold, stark, naked truth about who I am, and the sacrifices you sometimes have to make as woman. Here was an opportunity to force myself to not hide from what I look like and to see my own beauty mirrored back to me in the teary eyes of the women around me. The fact that I wear a prosthesis so I look "normal" makes it even more important that my body be acknowledged for what it really is.

Body image and the decision to not have reconstructive surgery are unquestionably the main challenges I continue to face daily in my head, heart and body, and this moment of throwing it all into the wind is one that I return to in awe of my own audacity again and again. The battles that I continue to fight in lesser and greater degrees as an Amazon are not ones of physical strength, but ones of love, compassion, forgiveness and openness to the changes that have come unrequested, but nevertheless in my best interest.

In the yoga class I attend several times a week one of my instructors begins with two questions: "What do you bring to the mat today? What do you need to heal?" Each time, to my unending surprise, the answer is, quite loudly, FORGIVENESS. And each time, I am brought to tears in that moment as if the concept had never occurred to me. Am I really still angry with my body for "betraying" me and getting cancer? Angry at it for taking so long to heal? Angry that it gained weight and lost the muscle I worked so hard to gain?

Angry that I am still in pain, still tired and still not done with it? Angry that I am far more vain then I ever would have guessed and not big enough to just GET OVER IT?

I am conflicted about how to feel about what has happened to me and its repercussions on my body. On one hand, there is no question that I have learned valuable things about who I am in the world, how to treat myself with more kindness and learn how to finally identify what I really wanted on a day to day basis. On the other hand, I resent the changes in my body, the changes in how I walk in the world, the multitude of emotional issues that creep their way out of my mouth over dinner conversation when I had no idea they even lived inside me. I resent the interruption to a life that was finally starting to go my way—kids out of the house, an amazing loving man, getting my debt under control and a career in front of me. How do you balance the conflict between being a better person at the expense of everything you used to look like, know, believe, and value as important?

Pema Chodron, a Buddhist nun whom I someday hope to tell how many times she has saved my life writes, "Loving-kindness—Maitri—towards ourselves doesn't mean getting rid of anything. Maitri means we can still be crazy after all these years. We can still be angry after all these years. The point is to not try to change ourselves—it is (about) befriending ourselves. The ground of practice is you or me or whoever we are right now, just as we are." I find myself holding both sides of the issue these days. I hold an acceptance and appreciation for what I have undergone and the strength, courage and tenacity that it took to get through it all. I hold a deep knowledge of myself as an incredibly beautiful and powerful soul with a deep connection to Spirit that resonates to those around me when I allow it to. I fully and wholeheartedly love and accept myself as I am right now. And yet, I also am so full of the opposite emotions-wishing cancer had never happened, angry that my life was uprooted, bitter that I am completely different than I was before cancer and insecure about how I look. This must be what Pema meant about the work of loving kindness—the ability to walk the tightrope of life with the discipline to not lean too far to one side or the other in order to stay whole. Instead of struggling with not struggling, perhaps I am learning to relax into it and accept the turmoil; to not judge myself harshly for the challenges I have faced and mistakes I have made and to maintain humility and grace in the presence of all I have accomplished. The idea is not that I need to forgive my body for its failure in getting cancer, but rather to forgive myself for viewing it with such animosity, for not loving all it has done for me and to see how beautiful it has always been—with one boob or two. I need to choose instead to view my body and its little dance with cancer with loving kindness, accepting both the positive AND the negative aspects as a part of a larger whole of beauty and light.

I have finally lost the weight I gained due to surgery, stress, inactivity and medication. There were things I liked about all the extra padding—the remaining boob was fluffier, I was filled out and the potential for me having more stomach fat to mold into a new boob should I decide to do reconstruction was a fabulous, if odd, bonus. But looking in the mirror and seeing a body that was so completely different from anything I had ever known—even if I wasn't looking at my chest—was difficult to say the least. As I started to think about reconstruction more, I realized that based on the past 40 years, I wasn't going to be happy with my body no matter what I did unless I changed myself inside . After all, now that I lost the weight I gained and became close to what I used to look like all I could see was how "damaged" I was. This even after I was easily back to the size 2 most women would kill for! I started to think... "hmmm, I wasn't loving my body when I had two boobs and was skinny and full of muscle and I wasn't loving my body when cancer took a breast and made me fight for my life. Now I am looking in the mirror and still am not loving my body because it doesn't look like the standard of beauty in the movies and tv. What makes me think that after I have 3-4 plastic surgeries I will love my body then?" The issue is not what my body looks like, but what is going on in my own head as my partner Neil has always told me. I called my plastic surgeon and had them remove me from the wait list and removed my name from the Victoria's Secret catalog mailing list as well.

My yoga teacher, John, and I had a conversation in which I told him that it was hard to send love to my body when such a large part of me was physically missing. "How do you love what exists AND what used to exist?" He replied that to send love to my missing breast and remaining chest area would take constant attention as there was no longer tissue there to hold the love I was sending. I would have to constantly and intentionally love what remained. I find this to be a very profound and deep practice. How do I love such a deep physical and emotional wound? And yet, to heal and to be a survivor, and not let the disease get the best of me, this is precisely what I must do. I must learn to love the power and strength and courage that it took to save my own life. Learn to love the fact that I am not the same person I was—internally or externally. Learn to love my scars and the differences in my physical being. And I must learn to love my sad little self on the days when it is brutally difficult to look in the mirror or be naked in front of my boyfriend because I feel like a freak. Remembering to send love to the parts of me that have suffered so greatly through surgery and radiation when it is all a blurred memory can be hard. It is necessary to tell myself the story again and again, to remind myself of how courageous I am and that the mirror shows a small portion of all that I am.

I can say the words, and most days I believe them, but many days remain when it feels like a boatload of crap I keep feeding myself to feel better. After all—that girl on the catalog cover that is probably 20 and looks 14 and has boobs that couldn't POSSIBLY be real and a flat stomach that means she must never eat IS actually what men like - right? Even the yoga magazines show buxom young women with low cut shirts bending over in positions that presents the fruit ripe for the picking. No man in their right mind fantasizes about a pasty, flabby 40 year old cancer survivor with one boob, scars from surgery and radiation and a butt that seems to be sliding down the back of her legs. How do I get past seeing myself as an object instead of as a whole being that is not loved or respected based on my appearance? In our media-based culture we are inundated with images of all that we are somehow "supposed" to be. But, it takes supreme effort to learn how to tell ourselves positive stories about who we actually are. Our tendency is to beat ourselves up for the things we are NOT and to not discuss the things we are because we seem to think that doing so makes us vain, conceited, arrogant or full of ourselves. So all we are left with is airbrushed, edited perfection that even the original people would not recognize. Telling our own story, in its honest wholeness is critical to our realizing how amazingly fabulous, courageous and beautiful we really are and to learn to live in the body we now have to live in.

I look and act years younger than I really am. I have been asked on dates by young men my own kids age and have taken pride in the fact that I turned heads (although I would never have admitted that to anyone). I am curvy and fit and have tattoos and thought that was largely what got me noticed and why people paid attention to me. Now, part of me wonders how I am supposed to reconcile what people see on the outside with what I know I look like under my clothes? Yet, I am more: I always speak my mind and am friendly and warm and adapt how I approach whoever I deal with based on their needs. My friends say I will flirt with a rock, much less people of both genders and all ages. I do my best to do my best, I grieve for the times when I fall short and I am hard on myself about the reasons why I do. I am loyal to a fault, brutally honest, and generous to those I care about. I work hard, take care of others before myself, am devoted to my loved ones and can be oddly and randomly reclusive. I am funny, sometimes smart and always completely dedicated to the things I choose to spend my time doing. I can be fierce and tough and a royal bitch when pushed too hard; I am intimately familiar with how far I will go to protect myself and my loved ones even though I would never discuss what I have had to do to survive. I love deeply, cry often and laugh easily. I get overtired and overwhelmed more than I would like to admit, am a huge softie, and often think that I am not a very good grown up. I have moments when I wonder how I got so smart, and more moments when I wonder if I will ever BE smart.

Many of these things are what I think make me a good person—the things I think make me beautiful. These are qualities I would love in another person and that I am learning to love in myself. Some of them are things I could do without and there is lots I am not proud of, but I am a work in progress and awareness is half the battle. We are a physical society and when I look at myself naked and face my flat chested right side with its scar I wonder... how do you SEE these positive qualities? How do you embody these things? I used to be a person that made a statement when I walked in a room. I had confidence and a presence. Now, I have attended the same yoga classes for months and I don't think one of my teachers even knows my name. How I walk in the world has completely changed. I don't NEED to be noticed anymore, which is funny since I didn't admit to myself that I needed to be noticed before. Is this because I don't think I am worthy of being noticed? I rather think that it is because I no longer need to prove that I AM. In a conversation with a male friend about a time before I had cancer, I jokingly said, "Oh, well, that was back when I cared about being sexy". His response was "well, not caring makes you more sexy than ever". Why as women do we spend so much time TRYING to be beautiful if, in the end, all that anyone really wants for us is to be who we are? So much wasted time, emotion and pain.

I am learning to accept and love THIS version of who I am. My body is an incredible, strong and awe-inspiring thing to me in all that it has done and put up with. I have climbed mountains and had babies. I have been strong and weak. I have done yoga, golfed and skied and made love. I have healed illness, rehabilitated injuries and been put through the rigors of having had surgery and it's follow up treatments to rid myself of cancer. And although I honor each woman's decision, plastic surgery to recreate a breast is not going to make me a better person, more socially acceptable or frankly more physically attractive. I will not be more feminine or wiser. I will just have two boobs instead of one and I will have another series of scars and months of recovery and the same issues about who I am that I have always had. The path of healing from the disease, and learning from it lies much deeper than that. The Buddhist beliefs in non-violence, loving what is and cultivating deep compassion for oneself as well as others, have led me to the daily work of loving and AC-CEPTING who I am and letting the beauty of that shine through in my actions. That is beauty you won't see in a Victoria's Secret catalog. It is a PRACTICE—it doesn't just happen and then I have "got it". But, the fact that I am even working on loving all that I am makes me, as my friend Ginny said to me one day "more beautiful now than ever before".

~ ~ ~

Back in the meadow the moment of silence seems to last forever and I wonder if I have made a huge mistake. But as I glance over at Carole who is also standing bare chested and crying next to me and feel the love and support of the other women who have claimed the path of Amazon behind me, I realize that I am never alone in fighting these battles. The support and love available to me are endless because the scars I bear are those of all women who struggle with being proud of all that they are and a tribute to all that we have accomplished. It is my fervent prayer my daughter will never have to worry about breast cancer and will always love herself for ALL that she is. As I claim Amazon, I stand next to all women, cancer thrivers or not, who may not yet be able to see how gorgeous they are in hopes that they may feel my compassion and love for their challenges. We are not alone in our struggles to love the skin we are in. It is work to remember—a practice—and I sometimes forget too... and that is why I tell this story.

# 33.
# We Learn From Each Other

## BY HEATHER MCCLURE CMF

*Heather D. McClure is a Certified Mastectomy Fit Specialist. In 1993, Heather, along with her friend, Diane Gesualdi, began looking for nurturing places to go and be fitted for bras, prostheses, and swim wear for women who had surgery for breast cancer. Together they became owners of the Profile Shop. Heather is also certified to fit lymphedema garments. Heather and Diane believe it is an honor to work with women both newly diagnosed and those who had surgery years ago. Heather is thankful that we all learn from each other as we navigate this journey. Heather and her husband, Gary, live in Bucks County, Pennsylvania. They have two grown children, a son and a daughter, a granddaughter, and five grandsons.*
*www.theprofileshop.com*

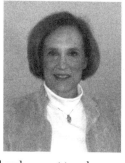

I meet the most wonderful women under the worst of circumstances. I am usually introduced to them right after they have been given the news that they have breast cancer. I have been that woman.

I was diagnosed with breast cancer in 1989 when I was 37 years old. Like most women, I didn't see it coming and I was totally unprepared. Truthfully, I don't think you can be prepared! I frequently say "it's the education you never wanted and you have to learn it as quickly and as thoroughly as you possibly can." My diagnosis came before the internet so my research was done in the library and doctors' offices, and I learned early on not to ask questions of anyone who was not in the medical field. Not that everyone and their mother didn't want to offer opinions, but they were almost always inappropriate, ill-advised, crazy or well-intentioned but unhelpful. (I would like to point out that the invention of the "world wide web" has simply made it easier for that many more people to offer their opinions, so just as much caution is needed.) It took me a few weeks, but, I finally learned to say "thank you for your concern, but my doctor and I have worked out a treatment plan and I have complete faith in what we have decided." I said it nicely but firmly so as not to leave room for any question. I would like to say that I believed every word in that sentence at that time, but that came much later. In fairness, I had many other people step forward who admitted that they had no idea what I was going through but they wanted to offer their love and support along with hugs, tears and many meals.

One of the most difficult things for me to come to terms with was the feeling that my own body had let me down. I was young, I exercised, my weight was where it was supposed to be, I nursed my babies—I followed the rules! Of course I cried, but the anger lasted much longer. I didn't smoke, I rarely drank alcohol—an occasional glass of wine, and I didn't even curse! (Boy did that change!) Looking back 20 years later I sometimes laugh and say maybe I needed to have some vices. The anger eventually led to a depression that really put me down. I felt that my life was totally out of control and I didn't know how to even begin to find my way back. I wanted my life back, but I wanted the life I had before breast cancer. I wanted to find my way back to normal.

I went through a period where I didn't recognize the woman who looked back at me in the mirror. It didn't have anything to do with how the surgery changed me physically, but the angry and victimized person staring at me was a complete stranger. I was not comfortable with myself and I am sure I was not the most pleasant company. When I went to church I kept praying for perspective because I sensed that if I could find that I might be able to dig myself out of the hole I was in.

I can be hard-headed (my children will love to see this in print!), so I fought real hard looking for that old tried and true normal that was buried in my head and calling my name. I was not kind to myself and was unrealistic with my expectations. I have since learned that healing takes place on more than one level; it is physical, emotional and spiritual. They are not mutually exclusive. I also learned that you can't set a timetable for healing—it happens when it is supposed to happen. The harder you fight your emotions and your own body's natural instincts, the longer it takes. It can take even longer to trust in that healing. There is a grieving process that needs to play out, and like any type of grieving, time helps. This is also where that trust in the treatment plan comes into play. The first year after diagnosis, every ache and twitch scares you. The next year is a little better. It takes a long time to trust again.

Approximately a year after my diagnosis, I started volunteering for The American Cancer Society's Reach to Recovery program. I found it to be cathartic working with women who were newly diagnosed. It also helped me to refocus my energy in a positive direction. In giving my time and compassion to these women I found my anger lifting. It took some time, but I finally realized that it was all right to let go of that memory of life before breast cancer and build a "new normal". My volunteer work branched out into other parts of The American Cancer Society, and then into support groups and women's groups.

The more I worked with women in the breast cancer community, the more I needed to. I became a spokesperson for the American Cancer Society and, in that capacity I was meeting incredible doctors, therapists, nurses and survivors; and all of them were focused on healing messages. It was like riding a wave of light and energy! I finally let go of the anger and refused to think of myself as a victim any more. A wonderful woman pointed out that I always referred to "my cancer"—she said "stop owning it!" She said the cancer was there and now it is gone, let it go! I learned Reiki and Theta Healing, both of which work with positive energy within your body. Positive energy! How could I not know about this? It's amazing what you can learn when you surround yourself with positive and uplifting people! That's a lesson everyone should learn without having to go through a life threatening illness.

There is a phrase I have come across frequently since I began working within the Breast Cancer Community – "Trust the Journey". I truly believe that the people you need will be right in front of you if you keep your heart and eyes open and trust the journey. Most of us start the journey kicking and fighting because we certainly didn't ask to join, but we can choose how we participate and who we take along as our companions. I can't stress enough how important it is to surround yourself with people who lift you up and to separate yourself from those who would hold you back or feed your fears. The same holds true with what you choose to read; there are many books and articles that will scare the socks off of you, but there are just as many that will give you hope and sustenance.

The last and possibly most important piece of my journey to thriving was becoming a Certified Mastectomy Fitter. My best friend was diagnosed three years after I was. She had both breasts removed within 18 months. I took her for her "fittings" for her prostheses and bras, but the experiences were awful. I put the word fittings in quotes because there was no fitting involved—we were given boxes with prostheses and a few bras and were told "try these". Together we decided that we could make that experience much better for other women. We did a lot of research, sought out the proper training, and after much searching found a bank that would lend money to two women who "wanted to sell bras". We went to the banks with a well thought out business plan, an explanation of what Breast Prostheses and pocketed bras were and how the insurance reimbursements and contracts worked. We were turned down by three banks but finally found a woman loan officer whose mother was a breast cancer survivor. She actually read the business plan, asked questions and fully supported us. Unbelievable! That was ten years ago, which brings me to the first paragraph where I said that I meet the most wonderful women under the worst of circumstances. It is my honor to work with them and to help them along their journey.

BreastCancerWellness.org

# 34.

# I Thrive by Giving Back

## BY WENDY MCCOOLE

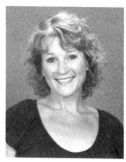

My name is Wendy McCoole and I was diagnosed with breast cancer in 2003 at the age of 42—the same age my mother was when she was first diagnosed 25 years earlier. Ironic. Things were VERY different for her—people didn't want to talk about breast cancer back then. When she went to the doctor's office... alone, because no one prepared her for what she might expect (so Dad stayed home)... the nurses wouldn't make eye contact with her after the doctor so matter-of-factly blurted out the news that she had breast cancer. They simply sent her home with nothing but an appointment card for the next week. I can't even imagine what was going through her mind as she sat in the parking lot shaking and sobbing. She refers to this as being a very dark time in her life.

I was more fortunate. I had a wonderful surgeon who canceled all his appointments to see me and my husband the afternoon that we learned of my cancer. Although I was terrified, I also had a calming sense about me that suggested I would be OK. And I was... and I am. So is Mom. And the beast even came back to visit her three more times—two more rounds of breast cancer and more recently a diagnosis of lung cancer. But we caught them all early and she's doing great. She's my hero.

What is SIMILAR about our collective journeys is our choosing to give back... to help make lives of breast cancer patients just a little bit better. Back in the late 70s, my Mom worked furiously—for ten years—to get a support group started at our local hospital. Why ten years? Because the doctors thought it was a crazy notion that people would want to talk about such a thing. They scoffed at her desire to provide an emotional outlet for breast cancer patients to talk and share and connect with others going through something similar.

In addition to the support group at her hospital, my mother was also very instrumental in co-founding the NH Breast Cancer Coalition. And more recently—in 2004 when I was going through my own bout with breast cancer—she was my BIGGEST supporter. I heard the pain in her voice when I told her over the phone that the lump was in fact breast cancer. I think somehow she may have thought she gave it to me. And I recall, as if it was yesterday, my then 18-year-old daughter saying, "I'm going to get this too, aren't I"? With a warm hug (and a lump in my throat) I comforted her and told her we would do whatever we could to make sure that didn't happen.

When I went through my treatments in 2004, I found it to be difficult keeping my friends and family updated as to how I was doing. I didn't want to bother them with email updates and repetitive phone calls. Conversely, often times it was uncomfortable for them to ask how I was doing. It was just a challenging situation for everyone involved... not just for me as the patient. So I decided to create a website called Bald Wendy where I would keep an online account of my latest treatments—photos and all. That way, people could visit the site at their leisure and read how I was doing.

I wrote about my treatments and how they made me feel. I kept a schedule on the site so people knew what to expect next. And although it was an emotional outlet for me, it was also a way for me to release some of those anxieties ... and to (somehow) find the humor in it all. Some of the stories I shared were quite funny—like when my nieces and nephew painted my head like an Easter egg and made me wash it so they could do it all over again! And when my daughter painted KICK ASS on my head just before the women's barbershop chorus that I direct was to take the stage at our regional competition. My head became quite a work of art!

I continued to write in my online journal and what happened soon after changed my life. At first, I recognized the entries in my guestbook—family, friends, co-workers—but suddenly there were notes from people I didn't know. They too were going through breast cancer... and they were afraid. They thanked me for sharing my story so openly and honestly because it helped them to not feel alone. It became clear to me that if my ONE story could touch that many people, imagine if we could create a community where ANYONE could write, read, share... and connect.

With the incredible support of my family, I left my corporate career as a marketing manager in 2005 and founded a non-profit organization called BreastCancerStories.org—an online support network where breast cancer patients and care givers can write, read and share their experiences with loved ones and with one another. It is somewhat like a blog site but what makes this community truly unique is that its visitors can search through the stories by age, location, type of treatment, and even lifestyle situations and find/connect with others going through a similar experience.

This has been a tremendous life changing experience for both of us, and now we get to share it and give back to others every day. Mom has been on our Board of Directors from the start and recently she's taken to doing some stand-up comedy about her breast cancer experiences! She jokes about having her prosthetic breast creeping up and hitting her in the chin, about standing up against a wall to make sure they are both even, and about how she is now a padiddle. Humor is absolutely the best medicine! And so is family—we are both so blessed.

# 35.

# Choices

## BY JANE MURPHY

*Jane Murphy has been married to her high school sweetheart for 27 years and she is a thriving mom of 4 grown children! Her New Year's Resolution was to come up with 2010 unique things to be grateful for in 2010 (She's at 1092)! She currently resides in upstate NY with her husband, 2 dogs and 4 cats.*

*"Courage is not the absence of fear. It is acting in spite of it."*
*–Mark Twain*

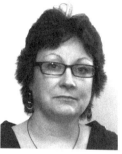

Every day we have choices to make—what to wear, what to eat. Most choices reflect our inner identities. However, when faced with what appear to be insurmountable obstacles, people often feel they have no choice. The truth is, we have a choice over almost everything.

In July 2008, my life was rolling along at a smooth, pleasant pace. My youngest child had just graduated high school, my husband and I had just celebrated our 25th wedding anniversary and I had just celebrated three years free from the bondage of prescription medication and alcohol dependence. It seemed like, after a number of years of struggle, everything in my life was falling into place.

Then, on August 8, 2008, I found a lump in my breast as I was dressing for bed. I didn't give it much thought, but called my doctor's office the next day and was fit into their schedule that same day. I told the doctor that I thought it was probably a clogged milk duct and she agreed. She gave me a prescription for an antibiotic, but ordered an urgent mammogram and ultrasound just to be on the safe side. It wasn't my first time having these tests, so when the radiologist came in after the tests were done and told me that I had to return two days later for a biopsy, I knew that it wasn't just a clogged milk duct. Still, I wasn't worried because both my mother and I had a history of fibrocystic breasts. I did start to worry, however, when I asked the radiologist who performed the biopsy what the possible diagnoses could be, and she told me she couldn't think of any diagnosis other than cancer. Now, I was worried. Two days later, my doctor called me at work and asked if I could go to her office when I was finished for the day. I knew doctor's didn't call patients after biopsies and ask to see them just to give them good news. I told her I could be there whenever she wanted me to be and she asked me to come right over. Within minutes, I was sitting next to my doctor being told I had breast cancer and that she had already scheduled an appointment for me with a surgeon. My life changed all in the timespan of a week.

Now I was faced with choices. Choices about what my treatment would be (although my options were limited). Choices about whom I should tell and how. And a choice about how I was going to let it affect my life. I had cancer, now what was I going to do about it? I could throw in the towel and give up right then and there. After all, life as I knew it was over. Things would never be the same for me and my family. But I chose not to take that route. I had cancer; I had no choice over that. I did have a choice whether I was going to be miserable and make the lives of those around me miserable as well.

I had a modified radical mastectomy on September 8. While I was in the hospital, the doctors and nurses commented on what an amazing attitude I had. They wished all of their patients had my attitude. At that point, my attitude was one of the few things I had a choice over. Why spend it wallowing in self-pity and negativity? Those emotions would not cure my cancer nor could they ease my pain. I decided that I was going to use my cancer diagnosis as a positive experience. My faith assures me that my life is in God's hands and it is not my place to question His motives.

Instead of dwelling on my treatments and their related side effects, I chose to make a gratitude list daily. Sometimes I write it down. Other times, it is just a mental note. But every day, I can find something to be grateful for. I have a roof over my head and food in my refrigerator. I have a loving and caring family and friends who are ready to walk this journey with me. My children are healthy and happy. I am able to get out of bed every day, dress myself and move freely about my house and about my country. I have access to top-rate medical care. I have a right to worship Who/What I choose where I choose.

The bottom line is, regardless of the circumstances, we all have choices. We can choose how we react to an unkind word or an unfortunate event. We can get hurt feelings or get angry which, in the long run, hurts no one but us. We can choose how we react to bad weather, clogged drains and broken shoe laces. Our choices can make or break us. Our choices affect us mind, body and spirit. None of us knows what lies ahead, but we can choose how we are going to handle each moment. I choose to handle my moments with grace, dignity, sobriety and gratitude and I hope to serve as an example to others.

# 36.

# Don't Spare the China

## BY BECKY OLSON

*Becky Olson is a professional speaker and author of "The Hat That Saved My Life." She is also the co-founder of Breast Friends, a national organization dedicated to helping women survive the trauma of cancer. Breast Friends is headquartered in Portland, OR.*
*olson.becky@comcast.net / www.beckyolson.com / www.breastfriends.com*

*"We cannot do great things on this earth. Only small things with great love."*
*–Mother Teresa*

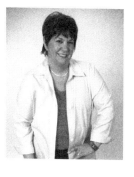

If you have ever helped a parent downsize, you know how difficult it is. My mom and her husband lived in their home for 35 years. The accumulation of stuff was incredible. When I helped them clean out their house to move to a very small two bedroom retirement home, it hurt to watch them pour over their items and make the tough decisions. But, there was a huge blessing for me - I came home with a box of treasures. Included in the box were four beautiful, fragile, etched glasses belonging to my Grandma. As I emptied the box, I took them carefully out of their wrappers, washed and hand dried them and put them in our cupboard with the "everyday" glasses.

When my husband saw what I was doing, he was pretty surprised to see where I was putting my newly inherited heirlooms and asked, "What are you doing?"

I responded, "These are my grandma's glasses. Aren't they beautiful?"

He said, "Yes, but don't you think you should put them in the china cabinet and save them for a special occasion?"

I reminded him, "Honey, I've had breast cancer three times. Today is a special occasion."

You guessed it. My husband's fear came to fruition. One day, as I was putting the glasses away, one fell out of my hand. It shattered into a million pieces. I was sad, for about a minute. I no longer had a set of four, but quickly realized that there are only two of us living in the house now, so with three remaining glass, I still had a spare!

Now, every morning when I open the cupboard, I think of my grandma. She died when I was about 12. I remember her, but didn't think of her often. Now, every day, I am reminded of the impact she had on my life. She came over from Europe through Ellis Island. Without her, and the struggles she endured, I wouldn't be here. It's part of her legacy to me.

As a survivor, I have spent a lot of time thinking about my legacy. I started evaluating things during my first battle with cancer in 1996. Like many of us who are hit in the face with our own mortality, the thoughts around how I will be remembered when I am gone began to come into play.

Being the top salesperson where I worked was foremost on my mind prior to my diagnosis. Working 12 to 14 hours a day to have a chance at climbing the corporate ladder had its benefits. It put money in my bank account, and plenty of it. It gave me recognition and a certain amount of freedom and job security. But I was unable to enjoy the rewards of my work. I never took time off. Vacations with the family were non-existent. I wasn't home to kiss my kids goodnight.

After my diagnosis, I was able to take some time off of work. I had nine months of chemotherapy to get through. The thought of being on the job—bald headed and with low energy was not something I wanted to do. Being in a commission sales job, you need to be in your best form. I knew I wouldn't be, so I took advantage of my employer's short term disability program and took six months off.

During my time off, I had a lot of time to reflect. I started to realize that those long, stressful, crazy days were making my employer rich, but would not make a difference to me or my family in the end. At the conclusion of my life, whenever that is, I didn't want people to say at my funeral, "She sure worked hard." I wanted my kids and my husband to have better memories than that.

As my benefits neared the end, I started thinking about my return to work. I didn't feel I could quit my job. My husband was working under contract for various companies, and as such, had no health insurance or benefits, and no steady income. But I did realize that it didn't have to be "all or nothing."

Many salespeople did well by being in the middle of the pack. I knew I had to find a way to be "okay" with doing the same. When I finally returned in November of 1996, those long days that I previously experienced gave way to eight-hour days so I could spend time with my family. I finally began to realize that it's not all about the money.

Those of us who have faced our mortality are fortunate. Life is short, and we are the ones lucky enough to know it. We get it. Things that we've been able to consider casually before become urgent. Things that were urgent no longer matter. Life and death is a fact, not a notion.

I was 43 years old when I learned about my first diagnosis. I was at the peak of my career. I was too busy to even schedule a routine mammogram. I had gone to my doctor for a routine physical, and she felt a lump. I told her it had been there for seven years and that I had a mammogram when it first appeared. I told her that they said it was fibrous tissue and it was nothing to worry about. Though I explained it to her, she insisted on a mammogram. She even made the appointment for me. I was so sure it was nothing to worry about that I had her schedule it for first thing in the morning so I could get on with my day.

I went to my appointment in my dressy blue "sales" suit. I had a calendar full of appointments that day. I couldn't wait to get started. Wow, did my life change that day. Somehow, over the seven years since I was given the "OK," my fibrous tissue developed into a tumor. In fact, over the next few days when I finally received my full diagnosis following a biopsy, we came to realize that my lump was actually a stage three cancerous tumor and already in my lymph nodes. My life flashed before my eyes. I was sure I was going to die.

My doctor gave me a 60% chance to survive past five years. Not the kind of news that makes a girl's day. I was in agony. I had five children. Some were still young and living at home. I was sure I wouldn't live to see them graduate from high school. I thought as many of us do, that my life, as I knew it, was over.

One night, early in my treatment, I sat down and made a list of things to do before I die. My own "Bucket List." I began to jot down all the things I had ever wanted to do. It was interesting to me to examine these items. Nothing on it was about making money or owning fancy cars. It was filled with everything I wanted to "do" or to "be." I had just started back to college three months before my diagnosis. Graduating from college suddenly became important. I figured that if I died with a diploma, people would at least think I was smart. I also thought I could accomplish it in five years. Having my list close at hand and staying in school gave me something outside my current circumstance to think about. Because I was able to take the time off of work, I was able to focus on school. I didn't have time to dwell on my fears. I began to feel better almost immediately.

I submitted to the "Previous Life Experience" program and was able to jumpstart my degree. I picked up 45 credits in the first four months by writing essays on what I had learned through my life experiences. Even with the jump start, it still took me seven years to graduate (I am so glad my doctor was wrong.)

Another desire on my list was to speak at graduation. I made my dream known to my advisor, and two weeks before graduation I got "the call." The dean of students invited me to be one of three student speakers. Finally, at age 50, I walked across the stage in my cap and gown and claimed my Bachelor's Degree in Communications from Marylhurst University. At my graduation party that night, my husband pulled a few musicians together and formed a band. They invited me to sing lead on "Oh Darling," by the Beatles, allowing me to accomplish a third goal; to sing lead with a band. I decided I better not quit my day job after that, but it was fun.

To this day, I continue to check things off my list. I found that by writing it down and telling someone else about my dreams, my desires, it's amazing what will happen.

When my husband saw my list for the first time, he realized that there were things he could help me with, like the band. I also wanted to spend time in Vermont with him at a bed and breakfast in the fall. He got on the internet, looked up flight information and had our trip booked shortly after he saw the list.

We've all heard throughout our lives that when we write it down, it begins to take shape. Whoever came up with that was right with one caveat: When you write it down, and share it with someone, it will begin to take shape. The key is to share it. High on my list was to someday own a cabin on a lake; I've wanted that my entire life. The idea of sitting on a deck and relaxing, away from the craziness of the city, was something I could embrace. In July 2010, we signed the papers on a very beautiful A-frame with a fantastic "half-million dollar view" of a lake. At night you can hear the roar of the ocean three miles away. Not extravagant or expensive, but perfect for us. In fact, I am writing portions of this story at the cabin. My husband knew that this was something I always wanted and he helped me with my dream. The key element about my list was to make sure I added something new for each thing I accomplished. I never want to finish it. When I checked off owning the cabin on the lake, I added, "Publish my next book by December 2011."

I found it was just as important to set dates for accomplishing my dreams. I haven't always made the exact time frame, like my graduation from college, but I ended up a lot closer. I heard this description once: A goal is simply a dream—with a deadline; without a deadline—it's just a wish. I knew I had to decide how I wanted to live my life - decide what kind of a person I wanted to be. I began to create little goals that I knew were reachable. By putting a deadline on each goal and taking baby steps towards each, eventually they would become reality.

Having the list has helped me to achieve things I never dreamed I would do. Driving fast in a car, as crazy as it sounds was a dream come true. In 2004, while going through chemo for my second battle, I went four laps around the Las Vegas International Raceway at 160mph while bald-headed.

If I can accomplish these things by writing them on a list, what more can I accomplish? What really matters in the end? With each diagnosis, my list became deeper and more meaningful. Now I am asking myself, "How do I want to be remembered when I die?" What do I really want people to remember about me?

An eye-opening exercise was to write my own eulogy. Not as it would read now, but how I would like it to read. When I first co-founded Breast Friends with my friend Sharon Henifin in 2000, we attended a class called, "Now is My Time." In that class, we had to pretend we were already successful with our visions, our dreams, and our lives.

It was quite revealing, and gave Sharon and me a chance to recognize the kind of women we wanted to be, and begin to work toward that goal. We laid out the blueprint for Breast Friends, and began our mission of helping women survive the trauma of breast cancer...one friend at a time. We worked part-time at our new non-profit, while continuing to work full-time at our regular jobs. Unfortunately, my day job was starting to pull me back in to longer hours than I wanted.

After my second diagnosis, I knew that I had to leave my job. I was still at the same company, but had moved into management. Being the top sales rep was no longer the issue, but I found myself getting sucked back into the everyday crisis that my reps now experienced. My schedule was inching back toward 10 to 12 hour days, and my stress was rising. I believed I was making myself sick, but I also thought I couldn't leave because I needed the company-provided health insurance to pay for the medical care I would need if I got cancer again. (How's that for crazy? To stay with a job that is killing me to be able to have health insurance to pay for the medical care I would need to fight a disease that my job may have caused. Yikes!!!)

Just prior to that second diagnosis, while playing the waiting game with the lab, I told my youngest son Micah, who was 19 years old at the time that the good news was if I had breast cancer again, I could take time off from work.

He said, "That's a little telling Mom, don't you think."

I said, "What do you mean?"

He responded, "You'd rather have breast cancer than go to work?"

He was right, and I was horrified. With the help of my financial planner, I began making an exit strategy and finally, one year later, I walked away and have never looked back. I quit a little sooner than I had intended though. It was one of those "heat of the moment" decisions. My husband was between jobs and no prospects on the horizon. I'm sure some saw it as crazy. When I called my husband and said, "Honey, guess what I did today."

He said, "What?"

I told him, "I quit my job!"

He said, "It's about time."

I left at the end of that day with a smile on my face. I had his support—something I needed so badly—and hope in my heart.

Three months after I left, my husband got a job with a company that had the same health insurance I'd walked away from. I maintained COBRA for five months while waiting to roll onto his insurance without skipping a beat. He's been there ever since. God is so good!

Many women who have thrived after their diagnosis say that getting breast cancer was a blessing. As I look back on my journey, I realize how my life has changed. I now spend my days helping other women with cancer through the work we do at Breast Friends.

I've never been happier, even though I was diagnosed, yet again, in 2009.

Even in my third battle, I learned something. As a professional speaker, my latest "opportunity" brought a new and even deeper level of sensitivity for my audience. It was the scariest of my three diagnoses. This cancer seemed resistant to the chemo. It was labeled as, "Consistent with metastatic disease." I live with the possibility that one day this disease may take my life... but not today!

Today, I can get out of bed. Today, I can function in life. Today, I can help someone through their journey. Lord willing, I pray that I will have many days like today.

I've met SO many women since my cancer diagnosis who have completely defied their prognosis. These are women, like Ann in Indiana, who were told they had a short time to live after being diagnosed with stage four breast cancer. That means it had gone into her vital organs and was no longer treated as just breast cancer. Her doctor "gave" her three months to live. A second opinion revealed the same. She was told to get her affairs in order. I met Ann 27 years later; healthy, strong and heading up a cancer organization. I met her when she hired me to speak at her annual luncheon in 2003.

I truly don't know what caused her to survive, so I can only guess. I'm guessing that Ann, like me and many others get up each day and say, "Not today!"

For me, I get out of bed and move through life "today" recognizing how special it is and refusing to lie down and wait for death to come. These ladies have significantly kicked their prognosis in the butt, and every day is a special occasion. For others not so fortunate, their disease may linger or even progress. But, many I've met get up as long as they can with the knowledge that their bodies will tell them when it is time to stop. What time is given to them in "months," often-times turns into "years." I can promise you, none of them "spare the china." They will break out those beautiful juice glasses. They will wear that special sweater they've been saving. They will visit Mt. Rushmore. I will never forget the cute redhead I met whose cancer had progressed from stage three to stage four. She told me, "I don't know if I have six months or six years, but whatever I have left, it's not going to suck!" She was a little spitfire and a true thriver.

By giving back to others, I found healing for myself. It's not easy sometimes. There are still days I can barely lift my head off the pillow. But there are good days too; days when I find humor and have the ability to laugh. I have been blessed in ways I could not have imagined before cancer. Sometimes I have to look for the blessings. But when I do, I find them. I have met people I never would have otherwise. I learned things about myself that I never knew, including how strong I am. I am still learning how to give back. Most of us will never be able to put our names on a hospital wing, or name a library after ourselves. But we can help others survive their journey through breast cancer by being there. By being the person who listens, the person that helps her laugh. We can be the person who inspires others by sharing our stories. Mother Teresa said, "It's not that we do great things. It's that we do small things with great love."

Consider writing a blog, or volunteering to help others through a local non-profit. If you can't volunteer, consider donating resources so they can carry on their work. Join a support group. Through our work at Breast Friends, Sharon and I have found that even if YOU don't need the support group, they might need YOU to inspire them.

Remember, there is a sisterhood out here. We are all in this together. And one more thing...Don't spare the china!

*(As of the submission of this story in August of 2010 —two scans following radiation for the third battle show the cancer is gone with no new tumors to report at this time. My next one is scheduled for later this month. We keep a close eye on it—but I try not to put demons where none exist.)*

# 37.
# Seeing Beauty

## BY JAN PING

*Jan Ping is an Emmy Winning Make Up Artist and currently is a make up artist for the Dr Phil Show and The Doctors TV Show. Her professional work also has included America's Got Talent, Tyra Banks Show, Stand Up to Cancer, Deal or No Deal, The Bold and the Beautiful, I Married a Princess, The Sharon Osbourne Show, the O'Reilly Factor, The Tonight Show, E! Entertainment, The Secret, Academy Awards, The Grammy's, The Emmy's, Country Music Awards, CBS Miss Universe Show and many others. Jan is also a national spokesperson for breast cancer empowerment.*
*jbping@yahoo.com*

*When I help others to see their real beauty,
it is such a healing moment for both them and me.*

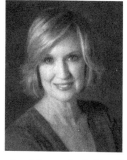

In December 2004, after having an abnormal mammogram, my doctor called. He instructed me to find a quiet place to talk and told me he was sorry but I had breast cancer.

I just stood still in the most surreal moment of my life. There I was, a single parent, waiting in the playground to pick up my young daughter from school and taking a call from my doctor telling me I had breast cancer. The sun was shining, children were playing, birds were singing, and all I could hear were the words 'breast cancer' and I immediately worried how this would affect my little girl's life.

The doctor continued talking about the cancer, but I had to stop him and ask "Am I going to live?" He said he couldn't answer my question and continued with the explanations of my medical results. I had to interrupt him again and asked him to think of me as someone that he loved and that person he loved had just been diagnosed with my type of breast cancer and that person asked him if she was going to live, what would he tell her? After a long moment of silence, he said softly "I think so". My reply was "Okay, I am going to go with I think so." It was then that my daughter, Alice, came running over to me wanting to know, "Mommy, Mommy what's wrong?"

We walked to the car so that I could have a quiet place to sit and talk with her. It was then that I looked into Alice's beautiful hazel eyes, reached for her little hands and told her I had cancer. While she was clinging to me, her tearful response was "No, Mommy, no". We both just sat there and cried. Then, all of a sudden I spoke to her with words from a different place of understanding, that place where I recognized my intuition and higher guiding forces were helping me in what to say to her next. "Alice, you are going to have to trust me.

I feel that I am supposed to do something with this and I think I am supposed go down this path. I am strong. You are going to have to trust me on this."

As I looked around, I started becoming aware of my surroundings again, feeling the sunshine again and hearing the children playing and the birds singing even though I realized once again my life was changing and that I too was going to have to trust. It didn't take long for me to see where this new path was leading me. It started unfolding when I went in to purchase a wig. My hair hadn't started falling out, but, nonetheless, I went in to find a wig so that I could be prepared if it did fall out. The moment I walked into the breast center wig shop, I recognized the lady that greeted me was a special lady. I wanted to know right away what her story was and what brought her to this place in her life of wanting to help women. I knew this was what I wanted to do, to help women in some way after they have been diagnosed with cancer, especially those diagnosed with breast cancer.

It was through this process of my life changing and the new me unfolding that I knew I wanted to enroll in dance classes. I asked myself what am I waiting for? I have danced all my life, but never considered myself a dancer. So I simply gave myself permission to take dancing lessons. Through the art of dance, I have learned that self expression is one of the greatest forms of beauty. Beauty comes through different genres and different areas in life. For me, dance is just one of the many forms of beauty and I love it. Dancing connects me to something more deeply within myself that I can't explain.

When I am twirling around in my dance steps, I am so in the moment of self expression and beauty that I feel more alive. It is so exhilarating. Through dance, I learned that not only does dance support our individual self expression, it supports connecting with our bodies, including the new parts of our new bodies. With each movement, I was encouraged to use my full range of motion by stretching and embracing. Dancing helped me to get in touch with everything that made me feel feminine again. I got to know me in a new way and to fall in love with my life. It is my hope that everyone touched by cancer comes to this place of self love. It's something I can't shut up about. For everyone to connect with whatever makes them feel more beautiful and more alive. If I were to give breast cancer survivors only one message, it would be to express their beauty in some way every day. It is one of the most powerful healing experiences they can do in their life.

Giving myself permission to take dance classes was one of the most amazing shifts in my life. It was one of the ways I started thriving after breast cancer. There is so much value in doing what you long to do. My mom, friends and clients tell me I have a new glow about me. They say even in the way that I hold myself reflects that I feel stronger, confident and more alive. Having been on both sides of the camera are very interesting experiences. In front, I remember the doubt, the concern of not being good enough, pretty enough, thin enough, character enough, and the list goes on and on. I think that is where my empathy and understanding come from. I remember feeling all of those unnecessary feelings that are so hard on our soul. Behind the camera, I can feel people. I have a strong sense of their insecurities having been there. I feel so fortunate to be able to help them shed those silly thoughts. Surviving breast cancer puts it all into perspective. All of the drama, confusion, and concern of such meaningless self talk becomes clear and is a very special gift in itself.

What brought me to this wonderful place in my life was listening to my inner guidance and just following it. As a professional make up artist, I have worked with some of the most beautiful celebrities in the world, but what I truly enjoy more is being with other breast cancer survivors and everyday women. When I help them see their real beauty, it is such a healing moment for both them and me.

My life has changed as a result of experiencing breast cancer and how I show up for the work that I do has changed as well. I feel alive when I am involved in the creative part of my job because I never know what each day will bring or who I will meet. I have a beautiful life and I am so grateful for my life and I say this every day.

# 38.
# You Suffer, You Survive, You Inspire

## BY PEGGIE SHERRY

*Pictured here is my sister Peggie D. Sherry. She is truly an inspiration and as her older sister I look up to her for what she has dedicated her life to. Peggie started out as an ordinary person with extraordinary ideas and God blessed her and gave her the courage and ability to fulfill her destiny. Peggie is the founder of Faces of Courage, http://www.facesofcourage.org an organization dedicated to providing life-enriching experiences for children and families touched by cancer. But what she also does is organize events that spread the important message of self-examination, early diagnosis, minority health disparities, treatment options and clinical trials as they spread the power of attitude, hope, courage and perseverance in the face of such adversary.*
*–Mardie Drolshagen Banks*

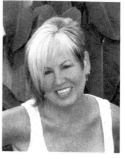

These words are taped to my computer screen reminding me each day that I must not forget the path. I have walked through the dark jungle of breast cancer, not once but twice. No one wants to hear the words, 'You have cancer'. In a moment those three little words, only 13 letters, forever change your life and the lives of those who love you and care for you. All of us thrivers have a terrible story of fear, indecision, hurt, loss, suffering and raw terror. So, to those who have not been diagnosed with cancer, I will spare you the gruesome details and only share with you that, since my cancer diagnoses, I have met the most amazing women who I now call my Sisters. Thrivers are a special breed. We look at the world through different eyes. We know that today is a gift that we were never promised and we know we are the lucky ones. Thrivers often make it their mission in life to stand at the end of the dark jungle path and hold a torch up to guide the newly diagnosed on the road to safe passage. These 'thrivers' are the ones who truly inspire.

How we get to where we are in life is an interesting journey filled with many twists and turns that we could never have expected. Someone once told me that my life's journey was like a mouse riding a leaf in the middle of a raging river, and that I had two choices: I could fight my way up the river (and get nowhere); or I could hold on tight and enjoy the ride. I choose to ride.

Many times newly diagnosed patients call me and ask, "When am I considered a survivor?" My answer (and I made this up) is that for the first two years you are a 'striver' you are striving to cope with the diagnosis; striving to put together your medical team; striving to understand what your insurance covers; striving to balance your family, job and illness;

striving to deal with antibiotics, pain killers, surgeries, chemo... and it's 150 different side effects, radiation, hair loss, and depression.

After two years, you have pretty much got it under control and you can yourself a **Sur**vivor. You are an excellent cancer patient, you make all your doctors appointments, never miss a scan, blood test and know all your counts (and whether they are in the ranges that they need to be). You can spell the type of chemo you have taken and can verbatim list all the drugs you are on and their interactions. Your hair is growing back... yup even your nose hair is coming back! As a survivor, you don't wake up everyday with the thought, "Oh, I have cancer." Sometimes you don't think about it for days on end. You have heard the doctor tell you that there is no sign of cancer and that he/she does not want to see you for six months to a year. You are elated for five whole seconds until you walk the door of the office and find yourself in a pit of quicksand... the quicksand of fear and uncertainty. When is it coming back? Where is it coming back? I need the doctors and nurses to monitor my vitals and protect me! My husband, children, coworkers and parents want the old me back... now. EVERYTHING looks different to me now. What do I do now?

One of the amazing twists and turns through the cancer journey was the realization that the people who came to my aid were not the people I expected to come and the ones who ran or hid or cried at the sight of me were the people I had called my dearest friends. Once the treatments and surgeries and regular doctors appointments are over I didn't know what to talk about any more. When people ask me how I am doing I say 'fine' or 'great' or 'wonderful' but I was not sure if it was true.

Over the next five years, many survivors struggle with failed marriages, loss of financial security, loss of jobs and loss of what was 'normal'. We take time to rethink what is important to us, setting new goals, putting one foot in front of another and taking one more step than we think we can. At five years out, you are definitely a thriver.

The thriver becomes comfortable in their own skin, appreciates their 'new normal' and faces each day with the understanding that this day is a gift and no one is guaranteed it. To me being a thriver means challenging myself each day. When you think about it, the three words "You have cancer" are just horrible. (The only words that I can think of that are more frightening are "Your child has cancer.")

Because you have survived those three life changing words I think it is important to judge everything you have been afraid of in the past to having heard those words. If you were/are afraid to fly... is that worse than hearing 'You have cancer?'... no. How about the fear of speaking in front of a large group of people... no. How about being embarrassed wearing last years style of clothes or shoes... hell no! Or having a bad hair day... hah, yeah right. Nothing should ever frighten you ever again. No fears baby.

When you truly embrace being a thriver, you hold close the reality that you have faced your mortality way before you expected to and are still here. Understanding you will never go back to being the person you where before cancer... you can't go back... so get over it. The one secret that Thrivers totally understand is that we have a new normal and I truly believe it is a better normal. Not that I would ever wish cancer on anyone, I can say that most all the Thrivers I know realize what a gift it is to be in this unique sisterhood. Our exceptional understanding of the journey cannot be understood by even those closest to us. But those who have walked down the breast cancer path understand completely.

We have each gone to hell, faced the devil, slapped him on the face and returned to talk about it. One of my favorite T-shirts reads, "Don't knock on hell's door. Ring the bell and run. He hates that."

Being a thriver is about living with attitude, the right attitude. Remember to honor yourself and your journey. You suffered, you survived and now you inspire... share your story.

# 39.

# I Didn't Want Anyone Else
# to Experience Loneliness

## BY WANDA SHUFORD–MIGUENES

My name is Wanda Shuford-Miguenes. I am a seven year breast cancer thriver. I reside in Tampa, Florida. I am a mother of two and a grandmother of four. I am the founder of Sisters Network of Tampa Bay; we are a National African-American Breast Cancer Survivorship Organization. I am also a volunteer for Reach to Recovery and a committee member of The Women of Color Cancer Camp.

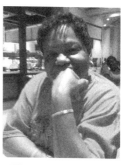

Being diagnosed with breast cancer was very devastating for me. Nine months prior, I had been diagnosed with kidney cancer. I started having pain in my right breast in February of 2003, I thought that the pain was because I ate too much chocolate during Valentine's Day. The pain continued for about a week. My first thought was that it couldn't be breast cancer because in November of 2002 I had a biopsy and was told that everything looked good and all I had to do was to keep a watch on it. Finally, I could not bear the pain anymore. I called my

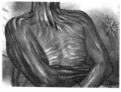

surgeon's office and made an appointment. He examined me and told me that I needed another biopsy to be on the safe side. From 1995-2002, I have had nine biopsies on my breasts. The biopsy results came back positive for breast cancer. On my return visit to the surgeon's office, he sat me down in his office and told me that I had breast cancer and that he would have to remove my breast. While the surgeon was talking to me, I couldn't understand anything he said, my mind was on how was I going to tell my husband this. All of the "what ifs" were going through my mind—what would he say, what if he can't handle this, what if this, and what if that.

So I didn't tell my husband for a while, I worked the 3-11 shift and by the time I got home from work he was already asleep, the mornings were the pits. I could not look him in the face with the fear of just breaking down crying. This went on for a week. I got a call from the doctor's office saying that my surgery had been scheduled and then real panic had set in. It was time to tell him. He usually called me before I went to work and that day I could not hold back the tears. I just started crying and couldn't stop. He asked what was wrong and I had to tell him. He was silent for a while and then told me everything would be okay. I went to work feeling as if my whole life was ending. The next morning he asked all the questions I knew he would—how long did I know and why I didn't tell him before now. I gave him all the what ifs and left the room.

Everything went fine with the surgery. I had a lot of pain and an infection. I don't take pain pills for the simple reason I am a recovering alcoholic and addict. When I had my left kidney removed, I overdosed on the pain pills that were given to me. So with the breast cancer I was not going that route. Tylenol was all I took. I slept on the couch for a week so that I would not bother him while he slept with me moaning from the pain. He would always tell me to come to bed but I wanted to be on the couch and suffer in silence.

Three years prior to my breast cancer, my husband had breast cancer. He always kept saying that he would not leave me because I was there for him. I had to go to my surgeon's office two times a week for about two weeks to have the fluid drained from my surgery site. I did not mind this at all because of the care that he gave me. I appreciated his care and how he helped me, something I had not had in my past as a child. He called and made my appointments for the Oncologist and the Plastic Surgeon.

I had four treatments of adriamycin and cytoxan (red devil). I lost my hair and refused to wear a wig. I tried wearing a wig but it was too hot for me. I never got sick just had to be isolated because my white counts kept being low. I had to wait almost a year before reconstruction which went okay too. On one of my visits to the Plastic Surgeon's office, I saw this lady sitting in the waiting room with this breast cancer bracelet on and I asked her where she got it. She introduced herself to me and told me that she was President and CEO of a organization called Faces of Courage and that she organizes and hosts day outings and camps for women and children diagnosed with cancer. They called her back to see the doctor, but, when she returned to the waiting room before leaving she handed me one of her business cards and said she would give me a call. About a week or two went by and she called to see if I could come by her office, she wanted to discuss something so the next day I went to her office. She told me that she wanted to have a camp for African-American women who have been diagnosed with cancer and she asked me if I would help. I said yes and we began recruiting women to help. We had the camp and it was a success. At the camp, I saw this lady from Orlando, Florida wearing a Sisters Network pin, I asked her what was Sisters Network and she told me what they did and how she started the Sisters Network in Orlando. She told me that I should start one in Tampa and I told her I would think about it. After thinking about it for a while, I called her to see what I had to do to start the process. I did everything she told me and, a month later, I started recruiting women to join the group.

I am glad I met Peggi Sherry at the Plastic Surgeon's office and glad I met Sherlean Lee at the camp. I felt that starting a chapter for African-American women facing breast cancer is what I needed to do because when I was going through breast cancer and I had no one to turn to. I didn't want anyone else to experience the loneliness that I had. I needed someone to talk with who had been through what I was going through. My family was very supportive but I felt as if something was missing. My husband found on the internet that the American Cancer Society had an on-line chat line for people going through cancer, I signed up for that and is where I go sometimes when I need some encouragement. No matter what time of the day or night someone is always on there.

Since starting the chapter in Tampa, I have met many women and men who have been diagnosed with breast cancer. I've gone many places and seen so many survivors and thrivers come together, we laugh together and we cry together. My "Thrivers" are Peggi Sherry, CEO and President of Faces of Courage and Sherlean Lee, President of Sisters Network Orlando, Florida. They took me under their wings and gave me the information I needed at the time and helped me so much. Because of them, I made it through a very hard time in my life. They helped give me something to look forward to. I now have a purpose.

*I would like to say thank you first to God, without Him, there would be no me. To my family for their love and understanding, to my Surgeon whom I will always admire, to my best friend Shirley from North Carolina for driving down to help me out for a couple of days, last to Mrs. Beverly Vote for giving me this opportunity to share my journey with others. I can be reached by e-mail at miguenes_22@msn.com.*

# 40.

# I Didn't Think I Could Ever Be Loved Again

## BY JUDY HAYS SPELLMANN

*Judy Hays Spellmann was born into a military family in 1942 in Nebraska and married a military man. She has lived in several states and the country of Turkey. She is the mother of two boys and three grandchildren, and recently, three step children. She is a graduate of Oklahoma State University and is a professional in the Child Development area currently teaching evening classes twice a week. She attends Church of Christ three times a week with all of her family. She volunteers weekly at a local hospital. Her hobby is travel, especially cruise ships, and spending time with her grandchildren and new husband. She can be contacted at jhays4@cox.net.*

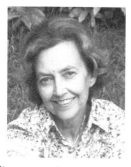

I have been cancer free 16 years. Breast cancer was prevalent in my family. Three aunts and my mother all had breast cancer. They were diagnosed with it in their latter years of life. I also had fibrocystic disease. In my 30s, I had had breast lumps identified in mammograms and biopsies showed them all benign. Yet, I still did not expect cancer at age 50. I have always looked to my Mother who died from colon cancer at age 81 as a source of strength in overcoming obstacles in my life and I did so during my challenges with breast cancer.

On April 15, l993, I noticed a dimpling on my right breast in the nipple area and I knew that was one of the signs of the disease. Not knowing what type of doctor to go to, I went to my OB/GYN. I described what I had found and he told me to go see a surgeon. I asked him who he would refer his wife to and, without hesitation, he gave me some names to check out for myself. I chose one and went with my husband. The doctor was very open and honest and truthful—which I liked. He scheduled a mammogram but the tumor did not show up! The doctor recommended that I have a biopsy to see if it was cancer or not. Results confirmed it was cancer—stage 3+. NOT good. I chose to have modified radical mastectomy on May 13, l993. Of the lymph nodes they removed, 11 out of 20 were positive. NOT good either. I then found a very well respected oncologist and underwent chemotherapy and radiation treatments. I lost all my hair and was in love with the toilet. Thank goodness medicines are much improved for nausea now! My husband was always supportive, comforting, and loving throughout this miserable time.

I chose not to have re-construction of the breast. It was too much unnecessary surgery for me. My husband, children and church family were VERY supportive of me throughout surgery; recovery; and my sickness. Without their support I don't think I could have had the strength to do the necessary things to get better. The memory of my Mother who was always so strong gave me the same strength. The chemo and radiation treatments made me very tired and weak and I sometimes felt death would be better. I stayed in the house most of the time and away from people—due to my immune system being "0". I wore scarves and a wig that looked so natural a lot of friends did not know I had lost my hair. It took a year for my hair to grow back. Two months after surgery, I was able to buy a prosthesis; it required a doctor's prescription. It looks natural under clothing and is very comfortable so I don't mind wearing it at all. I even wear special bathing suits. I returned to work one year after my surgery—I was so weak from the chemo! My check-ups since this have all been perfect! God took care of me!

I also learned to take better care of myself because of my body being compromised as a result of the surgery. It was thirteen years after my surgery that I was cleaning house and overexerted myself. I had put too much strain on my arm from which the lymph nodes were removed. That resulted in a stern lecture from my oncologist and lymphedema in my arm. I now wear a support sleeve except when sleeping or bathing.

Twelve years after my diagnosis of breast cancer, my husband was diagnosed with pancreatic cancer. He was 61 and lived 34 days. We had been married for 41 years. I was lost. He had helped me so much through my cancer and now there was nothing I could do to help him with his. Being a Christian family (Church of Christ), we turned to God and our friends and family for strength to get us through this again. I have always been in the military life, so I had been used to being alone from time to time—but this was entirely different. I finally got on my feet and returned to work and life went on. About three years ago, I thought and prayed A LOT. I did not know where I belonged even though I had lot of friends. I was lonely; so I was talked into the idea that it was okay to have men friends—nothing serious though—because of my surgery. I didn't think I could ever be a wife again, so friendship was fine. I went out with several men friends and they knew about my surgery and we were merely dinner and movie friends—someone to go out with and have a good time.

Almost two years ago, through church, I met a widower. I dreaded telling this new friend because I thought it would make him want to tell me good bye forever. But the first time we met he saw my medical bracelet and asked me about it. He surprised me by being accepting without reservation. It was a very open and honest meeting for both of us—not what I had expected—and it has been an open and honest relationship ever since. I don't know what would have happened if I had waited to tell him. His health seems perfect for our age—but we never know, do we? As it happened, he courted me for several months and we were married last summer at church with all our children present and happy for us. We feel blessed to have each other.

Ladies—I have learned a lot about cancer and life—through having people who really care about me—not what I look like. You can too! Four things I would suggest:

1. Find a surgeon you trust and an oncologist you trust to treat you
2. Lean on God, family and friends for support
3. Find someone who has gone through what you are dealing with
4. Be there for someone else who is going through what you have been through

# 41.
# The Journey for Healing My Emotions

## BY VICKI TASHMAN

*Vicki Tashman commanded all the resources and support available to her; she was a prime example of the active and pro-active patient. She interviewed different doctors, attended different support groups, signed up for different studies and never took "no"—or "I don't know"—for an answer. All this worked to her advantage and she is alive today because of it. Vicki created Pink-Link as a way to find another woman who had the same type of cancer, feeling the same side effects and process the same fears. Pink-Link is a free and confidential online searchable database of breast cancer patients and survivors on the Internet. The site can match women who're going through treatment simultaneously or can pair a patient with a survivor ... or both. Vicki lives in LA with her husband and two children. Her paternal grandmother died of breast cancer, and her mother is a survivor of nine years. www.pink-link.org*

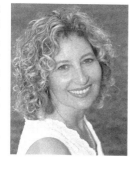

A lot of women can cry when they feel sad. I always got a big lump in my throat, but it stopped there. I never cried when I was sad or depressed. I never cried during a sad movie. I would have a big sore throat but never tears going down my cheeks. I can count on one hand the times I actually felt the tears, one of which was when our dog, Scarlett, was put to sleep and another was when I cried with my daughter after I was diagnosed with breast cancer.

When I was in treatment, I started seeing a therapist who insisted that I compartmentalized my feelings and couldn't label my emotions.

"But, I know when I'm happy, when I'm in love, when I'm sad," I said, "So, what do you mean?"

"Well, what are you feeling right this minute?" she responded.

"Nothing in particular," I said.

"Exactly my point."

So, that's when I began my "healing emotions" journey that has taken 6 years and counting. It started with trying to be present, in the moment, for life. Turns out (and I didn't know why I couldn't remember my childhood or past events), I was always thinking about the "next thing to accomplish." I was thinking about what I was doing next or tomorrow or the next day, but never what was happening at that particular moment. It felt so good to be able to regurgitate a conversation I had a couple of weeks prior, or when I had set a curfew for my son but he insisted that I never had. I felt like I was on my way!

I began to "check in" with myself. How was I feeling at that moment? Soon, I began to see some physical changes. When I got angry or became defensive, I felt the heat rising through my body. This was a new sensation for me and I began to notice it more. At first I didn't associate the feeling with the emotion, but soon began to get the hang of it. It took me about 5 years before I was able to recognize the feeling and emotion and act on it. I was actually able to use my voice and say, "I'm feeling defensive and I don't want to feel that way," or "I'm feeling very angry right now." I was so proud of myself!

As you can imagine, a lot of past issues have reared their ugly heads but, I'm taking it slow and getting used to the "new" me, my new "emotional" normal after breast cancer. I love this new me! I think it's made me a better parent, a better spouse, a better sister and a much better friend. It's helped me understand what the word "empathy" really means and to be able to use it in my breast cancer advocacy work and running the nonprofit I founded, Pink-Link.org.

# 42.

# Breast Cancer Made Me More Willing to Change

## BY YISA VAR

*Yisa Var is a graduate of University of Hawaii-Hilo with a Bachelor of Arts Degree in English and Communication. She began working as a midday radio personality in 1999 and has remained in the Classic Rock format on B97.1 FM / B93.1 FM for over 10 years. She is also a professional singer, voiceover artist, and a writer for Big Island Weekly with a focus on entertainment. Yisa is married to her college sweetheart and has two wonderful sons. She and her family actively participate in community plays, television shows and local movies. As a three-time breast cancer survivor and thriver, Yisa is active with the American Cancer Society as a volunteer for the Reach To Recovery program, she serves on their East Hawaii Advisory Council and she was chosen as a Hero of Hope for the class of 2011.*
*www.yisavar.com*

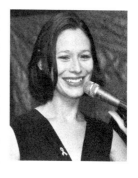

I am a firm believer that the person you are today was created by every experience you have had, good or bad; by every person you have liked, loved or lost; by every place you have been, be it near or far. It is the combination of the positive and the negative along with how you choose to react to each occurrence that defines you. Breast Cancer is one of those things that can be both negative and positive, sad and happy. It is life changing, but ultimately it has changed my life for the better! Every day it gets easier to tell my story of surviving and thriving and every time I tell it, I learn something new about myself and how this experience has enriched my life.

In 2005 BC (before cancer), I would describe myself as driven, hard working and goal oriented. I was working in a job that was not exactly my dream job and it kept me very stressed and away from my family a lot. When I wasn't working, I was performing in plays and with bands in order to build upon my local success in the entertainment industry. In other words, it was all about me! While changing into costume for a performance one day, I noticed an odd lump in my right breast. I was a little worried about the lump and asked a few friends to feel it to see if maybe it was all in my head. They all convinced me to have it looked at by a doctor, which I did. The first doctor told me it was a cyst. Three months later, another doctor told me it was just a bruise and I could follow up again in six months. That didn't feel like the right thing to do so I made an appointment for three months later. That appointment went the same as the rest concluding "probably benign findings," except this time, a few days after the ultrasound, the radiologist called and asked me to return for a biopsy.. After almost a year of hearing "it's probably nothing," I was a little confused, but followed through with the procedure. On April 17, 2006, at the age of 31, I was diagnosed with Stage II Invasive Ductal Carcinoma. The news came as a shock. No other family members or friends had gone through it so when I was given the diagnosis that I had the "C" word, I instantly thought that it was the beginning of the end. I was young and healthy, I had no family history of cancer and did not meet any of the risk factors. My only risk factor was being a woman. I was confused, angry and wondered why this was happening to me.

What did I do to deserve this? It was as if someone had pulled the rug out from under me. I didn't know which way was up anymore and had no clue what to do next. Then, that moment of clarity came and everything that truly mattered in my life instantly came into focus. I NEEDED TO BEAT CANCER! I left the doctor's office on a mission to find out all about the disease, how advanced it was and what I could do to beat it. Almost overnight, I became an expert on breast cancer, treatment options and pathology reports. I set forth on the path to take on the fight of and for my life.

Every question raced through my head, including ones that were very hard to consider. What did I do wrong to cause this? Was I going to die? How am I going to break this news to my sons? It was overwhelming and the only thing I could think to do was begin seeking answers. I spent six weeks doing my homework online, at doctor consultations and support groups. I found there were few treatment options available to me, not only as a young woman with breast cancer, but also as someone who lives in a small town with limited resources. I made the decision to travel out of town to seek a doctor that I felt would work with me to provide the treatment I wanted, with the best outcome. My options were a lumpectomy with radiation, removal of the right breast or a bilateral mastectomy. Chemotherapy was not necessary. I chose to undergo the most extreme treatment, which was a bilateral skin-sparing mastectomy, in the hope of avoiding any recurrence. I figured that my breasts had fed my two beautiful children when they were babies and had fulfilled their duty. If they were a body part I could survive without then it was worth the sacrifice. A year later, I had bilateral reconstruction and felt hopeful that this was my new beginning.

Eight months after reconstructive surgery, I discovered another lump in the same place that the tumor had been. The doctors again tried to write it off as scar tissue or maybe a faulty valve in the breast implant, but I was not so easily convinced this time. Although the doctor assured me that there was only a 1 percent chance of it being anything to worry about, I asked him to remove it. It was cancer again. I was 33. I wish I could say that was the end of it, but my story continues with a third breast cancer diagnosis in August 2010 at the age of 35, this time in the muscle of the chest wall. Even with the odds working against me, I continue to conquer, to learn, to grow and to thrive in the face of adversity.

I remember early on in my fight hearing other thrivers say that cancer was a blessing. That statement made me angry because I felt I was being forced to change everything I thought I knew and even sacrifice a body part to get rid of this awful disease. How could that possibly have an up side? Now, four years later, I understand. It is not that getting sick or having such a difficult situation thrust upon me and my family was a good thing. It is the people I met as a result, who offered a kind hug, a hot meal, a shoulder to cry on and an opportunity to find healing by telling my story and hearing theirs. I would have never had the chance to be so humbled by the good in the world if it weren't for cancer.

After facing cancer three times, I have learned so many amazing things about myself, about my family, and about the world in general. I have learned that as hard as it may be, it is okay to ask for help. For caregivers, being able to help with even the tiniest thing is a way for them to heal and cope. I've learned that sometimes the choices in life aren't easy, but deep down inside the right answers are there for you. You must allow that inner voice to be louder than any other. I've learned that the people in your life that truly matter will stick with you through thick and thin, and cancer. I've learned that attitude has a direct effect on how well you thrive during and after cancer and that keeping a sense of humor is a powerful coping mechanism. I have also learned that fighting cancer and winning can serve as a deep connection to others who have been or will be affected by cancer.

As a result of my battle, I have become very active in my community, advocating for women to take control of their personal health and make the decisions that they feel are right for them, rather than letting doctors tell them what to do. I find as many opportunities as I can to raise awareness about young women and breast cancer. I have become a volunteer for the American Cancer Society, serving on the East Hawaii Advisory Council, as a Reach to Recovery volunteer, and as a Hero of Hope Class of 2011. I participate in other events including Making Strides Against Breast Cancer and Yoga Unites, and I attend the annual Conference for Young Women Affected by Breast Cancer every year. I have also stepped out into my own community to speak about my experience and show first hand what it means to thrive. I am honored to serve as a positive example, proving there can be a happy, healthy and fulfilling life at the other end of this disease. I continue to sing and perform, not for fame and fortune, but to show my community that cancer cannot and will not slow me down! I also feel that through my survival, I am teaching my children that bad things do sometimes happen, but it is up to the individual to decide how they will handle it and what they will take away from that life experience.

Looking back on who I was BC and who I am now, I can honestly say I like this person so much better. She is strong, fearless and compassionate. She can find a reason to smile every day and takes the time to feel the sun on her face and the breeze in her hair. She only plans ahead for the truly necessary things, she doesn't stress over the little things, and she eats dessert first. She is no longer searching for who she is or what her greater purpose is.

Cancer came along and challenged everything I thought I knew. It forced many changes on me, but ultimately it made me become more willing to change. Now instead of taking things at face value, I question how to best accomplish the things I want to do and seek alternate ways to achieve personal success without compromising my happiness. My new definition of success is measured on a daily basis. If I can put my feet up at the end of the day knowing that I used each moment doing something that makes me feel happy and fulfilled, then I am exactly where I need to be. I know I am thriving! I am stronger and happier than I have ever been and I would not be the person I am today if it weren't for breast cancer.

# 43.

# I Learned to Advocate for Myself

## BY AUGUSTA WILLIAMS

*Augusta Williams RN MPH, has worked in the health care delivery system for more than 40 years as a staff nurse, supervisor and health care administrator. Ebony Magazine published her article entitled "How I Coped with the Number One Killer of Black Women." She has also written for Essence Magazine and recently The Breast Cancer Wellness Magazine. She is a 37 year volunteer for the American Cancer Society, and Past President of the Breast Cancer Action Group in Burlington, Vermont. Augusta is the recipient of many awards and in 1999 she was inducted into the Academy of Women Achievers by the YWCA of Boston Massachusetts. Augusta has written her biography, "Older than My Mother". Augusta is a 26 year bone cancer thriver and a 23 year breast cancer thriver. Augusta can be contacted at fgaleh@comcast.net.*

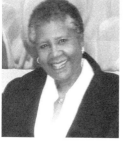

I began to thrive after receiving a phone call from the doctor stating "You have breast cancer." I did not like the doctor's approach. I did not ask myself "Why me?" But I did ask this question, "How do I move on with my life? Two answers came very clearly to me:

1. Empower myself with knowledge about breast cancer.
2. Learn to advocate for myself.

There are several things you should know about me. As a child growing up, I was a very passive person. I did not question any decisions made for me, nor did I speak up or out for myself. I was the little sweet kid on the block who was loved by every one.

The aforementioned behavior changed after I was diagnosed with breast cancer. I started to question and discuss with the doctors the treatment plan for me, choices available for me and obtaining a second opinion.

My second opinion was at one of the largest and respected hospitals in New York City. After talking with the doctor that day, he was able to answer all of my questions and I had confidence in what he told me. I was now ready for surgery because I had the answers I needed and I was being treated with dignity and respect. I made a unilateral decision to have a bilateral mastectomy.

I was a double F breast size like Dolly Parton. I was often referred to as the Ms Black Dolly Parton. I began to wonder how I would look because people knew me by my breasts and would see them coming before they saw the total me. My breasts were admired and envied by females and males couldn't keep their eyes off me. Now I realize my breasts do not define who I am. It's my total being.

My mother died when she was 50 years old from breast cancer. She also was a double

F breast size. She had one breast removed; the Halsted operation was performed in which all of the breast tissue was removed, the chest muscles and all the lymph nodes. I will never forget how my mother looked. She looked as she was severely deformed with a sunken chest wall, one large breast and an unsteady gait. I am sure my mother was not visited by a Reach for Recovery volunteer nor did she have access to any official publications. I have out lived my mother nearly 20 years with a diagnosis of breast cancer.

My second unilateral decision I made was to have reconstruction surgery. I did not want to be reconstructed to a double F breast, but to a C cup breast size. I began to think positive about myself after this decision. I now would be able to wear blouses that fastened in the front without pins to secure the closure. I have always wanted to wear a blazer coat but they would not completely fasten across my breast. No longer would everyone know what I ate at meals because the food would no longer be spilled on my chest. I would no longer have the pains in my shoulder from holding up a double F breast.

You should have seen me the morning of admissions to the hospital. My suit case was packed with pretty pajamas, satin pillow case, make up and perfume. I was proud of myself for making the decision I had made. I really felt good about my self and wanted the world to know it.

The hospital's protocol for admission was to call you the morning you were to be admitted to confirm that a bed was available that day. I received that call but it was not what I wanted to hear. Instead it was, "We do not have a bed for you, we can't admit you because you do not have insurance." I hit the panic buttons, and became very emotional, crying uncontrollably for a moment. I soon composed myself so that I could research why I didn't have insurance. Some one did not follow the protocol from transferring insurance from one job to another job. I needed help! I asked myself who could help me? First Lady Nancy Reagan came to my mind. She had experienced breast cancer and hopefully she could help. I called the White House and asked to speak with Nancy Reagan. The person responded by asking me "The President's wife? in a shocking tone of voice. I answered yes, her name is Nancy is it not? I was transferred to several people and then was assured that I would be admitted that day. I thanked them and sat quietly on my bed awaiting a phone call. The phone rang within minutes. "Augusta, this is the hospital calling and we have a bed for you."

From this experience, I've learned to go to the top when faced with what may seem like insurmountable situations. I have used this experience of going to the top in other situations, i.e. Sears, U S Postal Service and others.

After my surgery, I continued to advocate for myself. Funny being a registered nurse, I could not see how the doctor was going to remove two double F breasts without sinking my chest. I immediately called the nurse and requested her to call the doctor so he could explain the surgical procedure to me. The doctor came and explained the operative procedure very clearly for me and I was at peace. When my dressing on my chest was changed, I was so anxious to see the new area that I assisted the doctor in removing the bandage. The doctor looked me in the eye and said "You will have no problem dealing with this surgery."

I insisted on wearing my pajamas during my stay at the hospital. The reason is that the gowns that the hospital provide for patients make you look, think, and act sick. I encouraged others to do so and I went around with my nail polish and polished the finger nails of others. My room mate was very young and frightened by the diagnosis of breast cancer and so were her parents. The next morning after surgery, she wanted her hair shampooed. I told her, "Let's get up and shampoo your hair." She said no because we just had surgery. I told her that she had one good arm and I had one good arm, we could do it. Afterward we put on our makeup and pretty pajamas. Our family members came to visit and asked if our surgeries were canceled because we did not look sick.

A couple days after surgery, I was visited by a Reach to Recovery volunteer from the American Cancer Society. I was anxious to see a lady who had completely recovered. She was one of the most attractive ladies I have seen. She looked as if she had just stepped out of a Vogue Magazine. I made another unilateral decision to become a Reach for Recovery volunteer and to look as if I had just stepped out of a Vogue Magazine.

I met the most beautiful caring handsome man in the world and we married and both of us are extremely happy. You see, I am continuing to thrive.

I am now at a passage in my life where I am completely peaceful with myself and the diagnosis of breast cancer. The diagnosis or the experience does not consume my being. I am so very thankful for each day, the sun, rain, snow, cold weather and for the brave women I have met across the country.

I find myself with a mindset of sincerely caring, helping and sharing with others and above all to daily demonstrate my positive behavior, joy and love of life so that others will realize that breast cancer is not an automatic death sentence.

I will continue to thrive, to share, to inspire others, and to advocate for myself and for others.

# 44.
# Healing, Moment by Moment

## BY BEVERLY VOTE

*I was diagnosed with breast cancer in 1992 at a time when I was living my version of a great American dream life. I spent years learning how to work through feelings of devastation, overwhelm, fear, loneliness, and helplessness that followed the diagnosis. I publish The Breast Cancer Wellness Magazine in hopes of helping others move through their challenging times. In 2007 I was a recipient of the Yoplait Champion award. I am a Certified Healing Images Specialist and a Reiki Master. David, my husband of 39 years, and I live in Lebanon, MO. We have two children, Laurie and Brad, and five granddaughters, Lindsey, Brooke, Faithe, Mariah and Paige.*

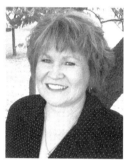

When breast cancer threatened my life again in 1994, the sequence of things which followed were much different than my first diagnosis of breast cancer. When I was first diagnosed, I listened best I could to the medical terminology, what was expected of me, what I needed to do and when I needed to be at the next medical appointment. I also sobbed in private, hid my fears the best I could, and prayed. In front of my family, friends and business associates, I pretended that my life would be just fine.

The oncologist and surgeon consistently warned me that it was high probability that my breast cancer would be aggressive and deadly when it returned, not if but when it returned. I had been having more frequent medical exams ever since the mastectomy and chemo because of this high probability and because of several medical misdiagnoses over a course of a year. My medical charts were flagged to pay close attention.

It was two years after my first diagnosis when I felt a new alarming lump in my remaining natural breast during my monthly self exam and I thought no, no, please no.

I first called the breast care center but they couldn't schedule me for weeks for a biopsy even though the assistant apologized profusely. I immediately called my oncologist next and was able to get an appointment the next morning. His findings were that I had three lumps, not one, and his advice was that I needed to see the surgeon right away.

I share this sequence because something greater was happening in my life that would not only save my life, it would change how I looked at my breast cancer experience and how I would look at my life.

The oncologist was able to schedule me that very day with the surgeon at 1:15. I was grateful for this, not only because this was a terrifying situation, but because I lived over an hour away from the medical facilities. My husband and I waited all afternoon to see the surgeon, from 1:15 to 5:15. We kept checking with the receptionist and asking when would I be next to see the surgeon since my appointment was at 1:15. At 5:15 the receptionist told us the surgeon had been called away to an emergency and that he could not see me.

What transpired in the following few moments was a turning point in my life. For the first time since being diagnosed with breast cancer, my husband became angry and started crying. He was so upset that I thought they were going to have to call their security officer. David had always remained very strong throughout everything up until that point. He seemed to manage the situation best by working hard or spending time in the woods. I could always tell when he had his sorting out time because it was there on his face when he returned home. We would hug tighter and closer without saying a word. We were both managing the best we could. So when he lost it in the surgeon's waiting room, this was surprising to me, and probably to him also. I didn't know what to do for him, because at that very moment that the receptionist told us the surgeon could not see me is a moment that I can only describe is that I felt like going out for ice cream.

When I have shared this with my close friends that I felt like going out for ice cream, many of them responded that I must have been in denial about the situation. No, I didn't feel like going out for ice cream because my husband was emotionally distraught. No, I didn't feel like going out for ice cream because I didn't have to face any bad news at that moment. What was happening to me was that I knew I wasn't going to have to go through the surgery and chemo routine again. How did I know this? I don't know, I just did, and the feeling itself was enough to celebrate. At the moment it didn't even enter my mind what was I going to do if I didn't have surgery. At the moment all I wanted to do was to let David know that I was really going to be okay. None of that pretend stuff, it was something that I felt and that I didn't understand, I just knew it. But David was too upset to hear me. We left the surgeon's office after making an appointment to see him the first thing the next morning. David insisted on driving us home even though I was more calm than he was. I was totally composed and at peace, and at that moment I didn't know why, I just was.

We finished the day by having a quiet evening and discussing that David would get his construction crews lined out first thing the next morning and then we would drive to the surgeon's office. I went to sleep in peace, still not knowing what was happening in my life.

The first thing the next morning before heading to the surgeon's office, I called a woman and asked her if she knew anyone who did hands on healing, and she told me of a person and gave me her phone number. Why I did this is beyond my understanding because up until then, I had never met or known anyone who had a hands on healing experience. I really didn't even know what this was, yet it was what I was verbalizing that I wanted.

We arrived at the surgeon's office at the appointed time, and the surgeon confirmed that I had three lumps to deal with. He advised he wanted me to have a current mammogram and a core biopsy before he performed surgery. I explained to my surgeon that I had already tried to make an appointment with the breast care center and that even with my chart that I couldn't get an appointment for many weeks. His response was that he had connections and that he would get me in right away, and for me to get dressed and his assistant would make the appointment for me. Yes, you guessed it, even the highly respected surgeon's office couldn't get clearance for me to have my health needs met medically.

Over the course of 19 days, I had 8 hands on healing treatments. I can tell you this, I took my friend Martina with me to the first treatment because I didn't know what to expect and I wanted her to be my extra eyes and ears. The "healer" told me what to expect following the treatments and what to do. She gave me no promises or guarantees. She told me I might be very tired after the first treatment and for me to be very gentle with myself during this time, and to drink lots of pure water to flush out the toxins from my body. She advised me that my body might smell during this time, even after bathing because toxins would be releasing from my body. On the third treatment, I could feel the shift happening in my breast, and not just my breast, but it was an overall body releasing experience. To say I was tired is an understatement. I could barely hold my head up. I have never been so tired in my life as I was after the first three treatments. I learned that this is how the body restores itself and that proper rest and proper sleep is vital for recovery.

Also during this time, I practiced visualization diligently every day. I made a connection with my body and "saw" the breast cancer leaving my body. I "saw" this in my mind every day for 19 days. Each of the eight times I laid on the healing table, I visualized my body healing and when I went to bed at night, I visualized this.

When it was finally time for my appointment with the breast care center for my mammogram and biopsy, I was not at all surprised when they couldn't find anything. Every technician in the center probed and probed my body to find the three lumps which had mysteriously disappeared. It turned out to be an all day experience. They were all very perplexed, and even called the surgeon's office to again fax over the diagram of where the lumps were located in my breast. I wasn't quite sure how I felt when all of the technicians and assistants formed a half circle around me asking what I had been doing. I answered that I had prayed a lot, which is an absolute truth, but I didn't include the hands on experiences because I didn't know how to explain it.

I share all of this strangeness with you to convey one message, that healing can happen in any given moment and that healing comes in many forms. Healing is a moment by moment experience, and that we build a healing momentum by building on the healing moments, one by one. Medicine has given us immeasurable knowledge, but the practice of medicine does not have all the answers. I have great respect for the medical community and for the professional and medical dedications to the mission of wellness. For me, I believe there is a higher wisdom for all of our lives and that medicine plays one aspect of the healing need. Each of us have a greater responsibility for our own health.

I believe that healing is possible for every woman diagnosed of breast cancer, and yes, even in the death process, healing occurs ~ perhaps the greatest healing of all.

Being aware and present in the moment has been the most profound resource for me to be a thriver. It is what saved my life. Had I ignored the feeling that I was going to be okay when breast cancer threatened me again, who is to say what would have been next in my life. I only know that I listened to that quiet knowing that came when I needed it and my life has never been the same since. I have been blessed beyond words since then with quiet wisdoms that continue to help me in my life and with my life purpose.

Anytime my life is not working and when I have pulled away from joy are the times that I have pulled away from the guiding forces in my life.

As publisher of the Breast Cancer Wellness magazine, I receive hundreds and hundreds of outcries from women facing breast cancer. There is a reason that the quote from Mother

Teresa "God speaks in the silence of the heart when we listen" is printed whenever we can. The reason is that we have to still ourselves, put aside our fears, and listen with the knowing that the right people or the right circumstance or the right message will be brought to each of us every day when we ask, and when we listen. The healing spirit resides in every one of us, we need to turn the connection on with full throttle. *{Mother Teresa's quote is included at the beginning of this book, right before the contents page}*

When I first ran across Mother Teresa's quote, it spoke to my heart with reassurance. Today when I feel troubled or challenged, I pause and still myself and listen in prayer mode so that I can know what is the best thing for me to do or say for the situation at hand; otherwise I find that my fears and my ego have their way, and that never serves me well.

I am alive and I thrive because of the connection to that power voice which is available to all of us; no one person has the exclusivity to it. By seeing the higher good in every experience, I move away from the victim mindset that at one time controlled my life. I have learned the world doesn't owe me a healing yet healing is available any moment I open myself up to it, which some times means moving away from my comfort zone and nonbelievers. And many times it as as simple as seeing what is right before me that I had closed myself off from seeing, due to fear and closed-minded thinking. Being a watchdog for my thoughts and who I surround myself with is my responsibility and is an ongoing practice.

Connecting to the healing moments in my life is what changes the channel in my mind, from victim, to surviving, to thriving. By continually training my mind to see the healing moments helps me to tune out the clutter of inconsequential fears, untruths, needless drama, nay sayers, and stagnant healing.

In closing, I invite you to claim every day who you are—you ARE a thriver! When you wash your face, look yourself in the mirror with compassion, conviction and strength and say your name, and claim out loud, "I am a Thriver!" Because you are! Let the world know who you are. When we do this on a daily basis, something inside of our being comes alive and resounds back with an inner vibrant YES.

Be connected, be a thriver!

I am Beverly Vote, I am a Thriver! And you are too! Let us be grateful.

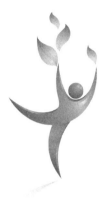

Thank you to all of the contributing friends in this book.
I thank you for your time, love, compassion and wisdom
that you have graciously and generously shared. I thank
you for your true desire to make a difference.

Thank you Stacie Marshall of Hill Design Company
for the beautiful design of the front cover and for your
painstaking hours of working on this project. I enjoy working
with you very much and I truly appreciate your creativity.

Thank you Jane Murphy for your generous help
in the final hours of the book.

# About Beverly Vote

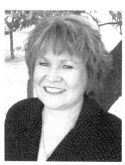

*Beverly Vote*

In 1992, Beverly Vote was diagnosed with breast cancer at the age of 38. Her personal life and professional career were thrown into a distraught tailspin. She learned that she had no point of reference for healing and no role model specific for breast cancer. Her fears seemed to control her experiences until she learned there were ways she could indeed empower herself.

In 2006, she created the Breast Cancer Wellness Magazine as a venue to remind women they are not powerless over breast cancer. The magazine is a quarterly, full color printed publication that goes directly to thousands of breast cancer patients and survivors in all 50 states as well as to several thousand mastectomy centers, breast cancer support groups, and breast cancer centers and events. In addition, the magazine is available online. The magazine was the 2007 recipient of the Don Ranly Publishers Award for Best Issue in its category and a contender for Best Article for the article Service, Strength, and Survival.

Beverly is a contributing writer for Chicken Soup for the Breast Cancer Survivor's Soul, Dancing with Fear: Tips and Wisdom from Breast Cancer Survivors and The Pink Prayer Book.

She was named 2007 Yoplait Champion, along with 24 other women and men from across the nation for their dedication in making a difference for breast cancer patients and survivors.

Prior to publishing, she owned and managed an insurance agency with the country's third largest carrier that was awarded multiple regional and national awards throughout her insurance career. Beverly's background includes event marketing and management.

She is the author of Breast Cancer 101: Lessons I Learned about Healing (release date November 1, 2011).

Beverly is a Certified Healing Images Specialist. She and her husband David live near Lebanon, Missouri. They have two grown children and five granddaughters.

www.breastcancerwellness.org
www.thriverscruise.com

**facebook**

BreastCancerWellness.org

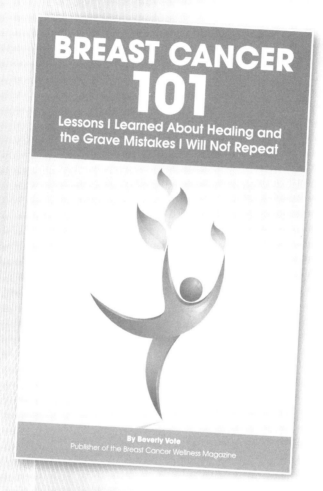

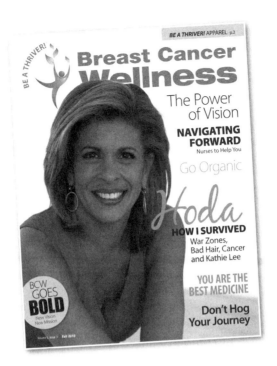

# Subscribe today!
## Only $12 for 1 full year

Name _____

Address _____

City _____ State _____ Zip _____

Email _____

❑  Yes! Sign me up for a year subscription (4 issues) of BCW Magazine.

❑  Check/Money Order Enclosed        ❑  Bill My Credit Card  [MasterCard] [VISA] [American Express]

CC #_____ Exp _____

**SEND TO**  Breast Cancer Wellness, P. O. Box 2040, Lebanon, MO  65536

<u>OR</u> **Subscribe online at www.BreastCancerWellness.org**